Fitness And Faith: Allies, Not Adversaries

Fitness And Faith: Allies, Not Adversaries

By

Dr. Bo Wagner

Word of His Mouth Publishers
Mooresboro, NC

All Scripture quotations are taken from the **King James Version** of the Bible.

ISBN: 978-1-941039-62-5
Printed in the United States of America
©2025 Dr. Bo Wagner

Word of His Mouth Publishers
Mooresboro, NC
www.wordofhismouth.com

Special thanks go out to several people for making this book a possibility that has become a reality. First, thanks (as is pretty much always the case) goes out to my dear bride, Dana. How many wives allow their husbands to turn their entire basement into a fully loaded gymnasium? And yet, mine did. Further, she has been my spotter on a bunch of my very heavy lifts and has yet to let me die; somehow, that is super-important to me.

Thanks also to my friend, Pastor Chris Hewett, for being a constant challenge to me in the area of fitness and for contributing several important videos to this project.

Thanks also to my friend, Wesley Morrison, for being a vocal supporter of the concept of fitness among believers and for contributing a section on intermittent fasting to this project.

Thanks also to my friend, Pastor Austin Vestrand, for challenging me by sending me screenshots of his daily runs and for contributing a section on running to this project.

Above all, thanks to my Lord and Savior, Jesus Christ, for giving me the health and durability to lift like a fiend; it may not seem like much of a gift to anyone else, but to me, it is worth more than gold.

Table of Contents

Introduction

Right off the bat, let me variously explain/apologize for the title of the book. There were definitely many other potential titles that I considered. Some of the real gems, I think, were these:

Bibles and Biceps

Turning Your Trailer Park Into A Temple

OhNoBesity! (Get it? Oh No, Obesity?)

Stop Digging Your Grave With A Spoon

Taking the FA(i)T(h) out of the Faith

Waddling Our Way To Heaven

A Grazing Mace How Sweet The Pound(cake)

Gems; definitely gems. In the end, though, I obviously settled on the more mature *Fitness And Faith: Allies, Not Adversaries*. I did this both because it accurately describes my philosophy that led to the writing of the book, and because my long-suffering bride, the Stiletto Spotter, threatened to drop a heavy weight on my head the next time I bench-pressed if I picked a juvenile-sounding title.

In all seriousness, fitness and faith really are allies, and I really am passionate about the subject. I have seen too many good people stop living long before they die, and then die when they could have lived for many years longer. I cringe every time I see people existing on two open handfuls of medication each day when most of their problems could have been headed off at the pass by changing the way they eat and the way they live.

In case you are curious (or even if you aren't), I am fifty-five years old as I write this book. That's right; the two strong, fit, mobile guys you see on the cover, both of which are me, are already fielding annoying phone calls from AARP asking if I am ready to join. And at fifty-five years old, I am on exactly zero medication.

Please understand, I am not knocking medicine or medical practitioners; they generally do a great service for humanity. I may one day need them, and my daughter, the nurse, will jab me with an IV needle in the middle of the night if I do not say nice things about them. And there are no guarantees concerning length of days; in spite of eating right and being a fitness nut, I could die tomorrow just like anyone else. But if I do, it will be *in spite of* the choices I have made regarding fitness, not because I have been lazy and careless and indulgent.

And almost anyone can make the same choices I have made. If you still eat, and if you can still move any body parts at all, you can make wise choices and improve your life; I do not currently know how to do eyelid bench presses, but if you need, I will figure it out for you.

But this book is about *fitness and faith*, not just fitness. You see, though what I will attempt to adequately show you in this book is good for anyone, I am especially gearing it toward Christians simply because they have often been taught that fitness is somehow a "worldly" or "carnal" thing to be avoided. And in that, the devil has won a great and easy victory. If his children stay healthy and live a long time while God's children are wheezing their way to glory (which, come to think of it, would also have made a pretty cool title for the book), then we are at a disadvantage of our own making.

So put down that 'nanner puddin for a while, my brothers and sisters, and let's get ready to change our lives for the better.

Dr. Bo Wagner

Section One
Foundational Issues

Chapter One
The Elephant in the (Church) Room

It was a funeral; I cannot stand them, but all of us will have one eventually if Jesus tarries His coming long enough. I was not the preacher that day; I was just there to pay my respects.

As I walked into the large and lovely foyer of the church, a church that I knew reasonably well, I overheard two men talking. I knew them; they were both deacons in that church. One would think, then, that these venerable men would know the Bible and be accurate in how they handle it, right?

Nope.

"Well, the Bible does say exercise don't do no good," the first one said with utter certainty. The second merely nodded in assent and said, "Yup."

I wish, oh, how I wish such ignorance of the subject was an aberration! But I am well aware of the fact that, far from being an aberration, it is actually a fairly commonly held viewpoint among the church crowd, and I mean among the church crowd everywhere. Part of this is likely because of the rotund reverends who love to make a joke about their fallen arches that they got from the golden arches. Part of it, though, is from an honest misunderstanding of a portion of Scripture:

1 Timothy 4:7 *But refuse profane and old wives' fables, and exercise thyself rather unto godliness. 8 For bodily exercise profiteth little: but godliness is profitable unto all things, having promise of the life that now is, and of that which is to come.*

And there it is: *bodily exercise profiteth little.* Behold, the Christian's "Get Out Of The Gym Free" card! Now we have permission to lie on the couch watching television while eating ice cream out of a bucket each night!

Not so fast, chunk-muffin. Yes, those words are, in fact, the inspired words of God. But in the words of that legendary theologian, Inigo Montoya, "You keep using those words; I do not think they mean what you think they mean."

The two uses of exercise do refer to physical exertion; they both come from words that we get our English words *gymnasium* and *gymnastics* from. But it is that word *little* that we really ought to look at for a moment. It is from the word *oligos*, and it means *a small amount*. And do you know what a small amount is not? It is not *nothing*. It is not "exercise don't do no good."

Furthermore, please notice that Paul told Timothy to refuse something, *but exercise was not that something*. Profane and old wives' fables were that something, which Paul then contrasted with spiritual exercise. See, those two things are opposites; doing spiritual exercises like reading your Bible and studying and praying will keep you from getting bogged down in ridiculous old wives' tales, and vice versa. And it is in that context that Paul then says *For bodily exercise profiteth little: but godliness is profitable unto all things, having promise of the life that now is, and of that which is to come.* So this passage is not an attack on physical exercise; it is an attack on the fables and other ridiculous things that would keep us from spiritual exercise. The fact that bodily exercise only profits a little while spiritual exercise profits in all things was Paul's way of motivating Timothy to do more spiritual exercise. But it was not, at all, a command or even a suggestion that a Christian should not exercise. And any Christian that tries to take it that way may want to know one teeeeeeeeeny little thing about Paul, the man who wrote these words:

He walked somewhere around ten thousand miles while on his three missionary journeys.

So, if you want to use his words as an excuse not to ever exercise, I am perfectly fine with that, as long as you, too, walk ten thousand miles or so in just a few years' time!

And now, let me give you all of the other passages the critics of fit-Christianity normally use to prove their point:

That's it. That one verse was the entire list. So, on the strength of one verse whose context is completely ignored, and in opposition to the myriad of verses that teach how beneficial it is to eat right and be physically active, Christians will be diabetes deacons and pop-the-buttons pastors and morbidly obese members while congratulating themselves on their imagined spirituality.

Such things ought not to be. That body you are riding around in each day was bought by another some time back:

1 Corinthians 6:19 *What? know ye not that **your body** is the temple of the Holy Ghost which is in you, which ye have of God, and ye are not your own?* **20** *For ye are bought with a price: therefore glorify God in **your body**, and in your spirit, which are God's.*

The price God paid for you was the death of His Son on Calvary; that purchase price was not just for your soul; this verse specifically states that it was for your body as well. And it was bought as a temple for the Holy Ghost Himself, the third member of the Trinity, to dwell in on this earth! No wonder Paul commanded that we therefore glorify God in our bodies even before telling us to glorify Him in our spirits. What Christians often do to their bodies is nothing short of vandalism of God's property.

15

Think about it; you would never key God's car or take a baseball bat to His mailbox, so why would you think it is okay to wreck His temple with lard and laziness?

Throughout Scripture, God draws a clear distinction between what He finds acceptable in the body and what He finds reprehensible in the body. Here is a tiny sampling of the acceptable:

Leviticus 16:21 *And Aaron shall lay both his hands upon the head of the live goat, and confess over him all the iniquities of the children of Israel, and all their transgressions in all their sins, putting them upon the head of the goat, and shall send him away by the hand of a* <u>*fit man*</u> *into the wilderness:*

Judges 6:12 *And the angel of the LORD appeared unto him, and said unto him, The LORD is with thee, thou* <u>*mighty man*</u> *of valour.*

Luke 11:21 *When a* <u>*strong man*</u> *armed keepeth his palace, his goods are in peace:*

1 Chronicles 12:8 *And of the Gadites there separated themselves unto David into the hold to the wilderness men of* <u>*might*</u>*, and men of war* <u>*fit for the battle*</u>*, that could handle shield and buckler, whose faces were like the faces of lions, and were as* <u>*swift*</u> *as the roes upon the mountains;*

1 Samuel 9:1 *Now there was a man of Benjamin, whose name was Kish, the son of Abiel, the son of Zeror, the son of Bechorath, the son of Aphiah, a Benjamite, a mighty* <u>*man of power*</u>*.*

Are you seeing the common thread? Fit, mighty, strong, swift, powerful. I could print literally hundreds of verses giving the same idea; God prized people who were as fit and capable as they could be. And not just men, friend, not just men:

Judges 4:17 *Howbeit Sisera fled away on his feet to the tent of Jael the wife of Heber the Kenite: for there was peace between Jabin the king of Hazor and the house of Heber the Kenite.* **18** *And Jael went out to meet Sisera, and said unto him,*

16

Turn in, my lord, turn in to me; fear not. And when he had turned in unto her into the tent, she covered him with a mantle. 19 And he said unto her, Give me, I pray thee, a little water to drink; for I am thirsty. And she opened a bottle of milk, and gave him drink, and covered him. 20 Again he said unto her, Stand in the door of the tent, and it shall be, when any man doth come and enquire of thee, and say, Is there any man here? that thou shalt say, No. 21 Then Jael Heber's wife took a nail of the tent, and took an hammer in her hand, and went softly unto him, and smote the nail into his temples, and fastened it into the ground: for he was fast asleep and weary. So he died. 22 And, behold, as Barak pursued Sisera, Jael came out to meet him, and said unto him, Come, and I will shew thee the man whom thou seekest. And when he came into her tent, behold, Sisera lay dead, and the nail was in his temples.

Israel was at war, and public enemy number one was getting away. If he did, he would be back with more men and more trouble. Unfortunately for him, he happened to stop in at the house of a little woman named Jael, otherwise known as Thorina, who whipped out her hammer and whacked a giant nail through his head.

Tough chick, that one. Here was another one like her:

Judges 9:52 *And Abimelech came unto the tower, and fought against it, and went hard unto the door of the tower to burn it with fire. 53 And a certain woman cast a piece of a millstone upon Abimelech's head, and all to brake his skull.*

I love the wording: *and all to brake his skull*. The unnamed woman saved the day by chucking a huge rock down on the head of the guy trying to burn them all to death.

By contrast, here is just a bit of what God finds reprehensible:

Proverbs 26:14 *As the door turneth upon his hinges, so doth the <u>slothful</u> upon his bed.*

Proverbs 6:9 *How long wilt thou sleep, O <u>sluggard</u>? when wilt thou arise out of thy sleep?*

17

Deuteronomy 21:20 *And they shall say unto the elders of his city, This our son is stubborn and rebellious, he will not obey our voice; he is a __glutton__, and a drunkard.*

Proverbs 23:2 *And put a knife to thy throat, if thou be a man __given to appetite__.*

Slothful, sluggard, glutton, given to appetite. Those four phrases all by themselves paint a fairly accurate picture of what we see in much of Christianity today! And that is even without the sickening account of Eglon:

Judges 3:17 *And he brought the present unto Eglon king of Moab: and Eglon was __a very fat man__. 18 And when he had made an end to offer the present, he sent away the people that bare the present. 19 But he himself turned again from the quarries that were by Gilgal, and said, I have a secret errand unto thee, O king: who said, Keep silence. And all that stood by him went out from him. 20 And Ehud came unto him; and he was sitting in a summer parlour, which he had for himself alone. And Ehud said, I have a message from God unto thee. And he arose out of his seat. 21 And Ehud put forth his left hand, and took the dagger from his right thigh, and thrust it into his belly: 22 __And the haft also went in after the blade; and the fat closed upon the blade, so that he could not draw the dagger out of his belly__; and the dirt came out.*

Ewwwwww.

Are you kind of getting the picture? In summary form, "Fit and active: good. Fat and lazy: bad."

In case you are wondering, yes, I am going to teach you what I know about working out and eating right. I am even going to provide QR codes for you to watch specific how-to videos of the exercises I describe. But this chapter and a few others really do need to come first, simply because when it comes to this subject, bad philosophy makes for big pattooties. If you think the Bible is against you eating right and working out, you will eat like a moose and live a sedentary, lazy life. But if you understand that God gave you one life, one body, and that it is a gift from His hand, and that you do not get another, you will be much more inclined to do the things necessary to change your body and your life.

You can do this.

Chapter Two
A Matter of Testimony

His ginormous head looked like a massive tomato that could pop at any second. His chin and his neck were like Yoda and the force: they had become one. The preacher was a sweat-slinging, gasping-for-breath, stroke waiting to happen as he screamed about drinking and fornicating and drugs (all of which I am against, by the way) and pounded his easily four-hundred-plus pound self across the platform.

And then it happened; as he finally gasped for a long breath, in those seconds of silence, I heard a voice near me that said, "Maybe he ought to learn how to push away from the table before he hammers on everybody else's sins."

Ouch; if that preacher had heard that, and if it had managed to penetrate all of the blubber, it could definitely have hurt his feelings.

We were at a pizza place some years ago, one of those that you can either order from the menu or eat off the buffet. A preacher and his wife walked in; we knew them from a different place a few years back. I am not exaggerating when I say that both were well over 400 pounds. They made their way to a booth and then realized neither could fit on their side, nor would there have been room for their car-sized cabooses if they had tried to sit side by side. So they pushed the bench back on each side, thereby pushing the other side of the bench into the table on either side of them; the two of them, by themselves, thus managed to take up three booths. And then they loaded down their plates time and again, a veritable Mount Food-Ji that they gorged on all the while we were there.

Pray tell, how can any Christian, let alone any preacher, show such a lack of temperance and still expect to have any credibility when they preach on anything concerning the flesh? Yes, I well understand that there are physical conditions and maladies that sometimes make it difficult for people to be very physically active; I am not ripping into people in such cases at all. But when obesity comes through the volume and content of what is put into the mouth, combined with a refusal to be active in some way, even though you could, then I do not hesitate to call it what it is:

Sin.

You do remember, I trust, the verse on gluttony I gave you earlier? Here it is again, with another one to accompany it:

Deuteronomy 21:20 *And they shall say unto the elders of his city, This our son is stubborn and rebellious, he will not obey our voice; he is a glutton, and a drunkard. 21 And all the men of his city shall stone him with stones, that he die: so shalt thou put evil away from among you; and all Israel shall hear, and fear.*

There is also the passage from the New Testament I gave you about the ownership of the body, plus another one that also deals with that subject:

1 Corinthians 6:19 *What? know ye not that your body is the temple of the Holy Ghost which is in you, which ye have of God, and ye are not your own? 20 For ye are bought with a price: therefore glorify God in your body, and in your spirit, which are God's.*

1 Corinthians 3:17 *If any man defile the temple of God, him shall God destroy; for the temple of God is holy, which temple ye are.*

You cannot wreck God's property through laziness and poor choices and rightly call it anything other than sin. But as the title of this chapter states, this is also a matter of testimony. When people see Christians sin with their favorite combo, the McLard with a biggie side of Lazy, it damages our testimony before a world that needs us to be pure in the matter of testimony. Look at what Paul called all of us:

2 Corinthians 5:20 *Now then we are ambassadors for Christ, as though God did beseech you by us: we pray you in Christ's stead, be ye reconciled to God.*

We are ambassadors for Christ; we are the representatives of heaven and heaven's King on this earth. When they see us, what they see is supposed to make them think of the God we represent. This matter of fitness really does go along with faith, especially when it comes to our testimony.

Can this get wildly out of balance? Certainly; there is nothing we goofy humans cannot get wrong, it seems. It is, therefore, entirely possible for a Christian to get so fixated on fitness, so obsessed with how he or she looks, so consumed with counting every calorie and lifting every possible weight, and posting so many poses that they become functional polytheists with themselves at the top of their pantheon of gods. But while that is a possibility, think about this and be honest: as you look around at the average Christian church congregation, does that seem to be the main problem? Or does the exact opposite seem to be the main problem? My anecdotal evaluation is that for every Christian who has taken the fitness thing way too far, there are ten thousand whose only exercise is the chicken-leg curl and whose theme song for going to heaven should honestly be "Swing Wide The Gates."

So get fit: it really is a matter of testimony.

You can do this!

Chapter Three
Don't You Dare Say It!

Someone, I cannot remember who, put me onto a fairly entertaining movie franchise a few years ago. I will tell you up front that we always use a filter of some kind to watch any television or movies; no Christian should pour filth into his head and heart through his ears or eyes. We use a filter that screens out any bad language and any nudity for any movie we watch. That disclaimer given, with something like Clear Play or TV Guardian or the like, we personally find the John Wick movies to be fun.

For those who do not know, John Wick is a fictional assassin, the very best in the world. The movies are incredibly over-the-top; I think the only thing he does not use to kill someone is a cheese omelet. But it is that over-the-top nature that makes them fun to begin with. John Wick seems to be able to kill anyone with anything, and even after he is "dead," we aren't really sure that he is dead; that question was left very much open.

But if John Wick were real, he would be a pitiful second place to the greatest assassin the world has ever known. There is nowhere this assassin has not infiltrated at one point or another, and very few he cannot ultimately destroy.

His name is "I Don't Have Time."

I lost a very dear friend a few years ago. Making matters all the worse, he was not just a dear friend to me; he was a dear friend and a godly mentor to all three of my children. In his youth, he had been incredibly active and athletic. Like me, God called him into the ministry. And as far as ministers go, he was one of the truly good ones. He had a heart for God, a heart for the Word of God, and a heart for people. And because of his big heart, he gave of himself, and here is the key in this discussion, he gave of his time to the ministry.

In fact, he overgave of that precious commodity. In specific, all of the time that he used to give to being active and athletic and fit was channeled into the ministry. His weight ballooned, and he ended up with high blood pressure. And yet, even that warning sign did not deter him; he continued to plow ahead both into the ministry and into the poor eating habits and lifestyle choices he was making to facilitate that ministry.

I will never forget the day the call came in. I was in one of our Sunday school rooms at the church on my hands and knees, not praying, laying carpet tiles. I have always loved hard work; it is one of the ways I try to stay active.

When I answered the phone, it was one of my frantic children; my friend, their mentor, had a heart attack and was on his way to the hospital. A few hours later, we got the word that he did not make it. Only later did we learn that he had been having difficulty for a few weeks, but did not go to the hospital because, in his own words, "I don't have the time."

I wish he had taken the time. I wish he had taken the time (for years!) to eat right, exercise, and go to the doctor when needed. This was not a bad guy; he was the best of the best, a gem of humanity, genuinely one of the nicest people Earth will ever be blessed with.

His mistake is not uncommon. If I had a dollar for every time someone told me they do not have time to work out and eat right, I would have enough to rent a large billboard by a major U.S. Interstate with the words "Stop Saying That!" emblazoned on it.

You do, in fact, have time. Everyone does.

Have you ever considered the foolish absurdity of the statement "I don't have time?" It is almost as if some people have twenty-eight or twenty-nine hours a day with which to work, while others have somehow been shortchanged and only have sixteen or seventeen hours in that same day. But the day is determined by the rotation of the earth, which takes within milliseconds of exactly twenty-four hours every single day, as regular as... clockwork.

Everyone has time; the issue is how we allocate it.

Now, before someone says something snarky like, "That's easy for you to say; you're just a pastor," please allow me to inform you that I am actually a pastor/evangelist/author/ newspaper columnist/high school Bible teacher, along with being the chief plumber/electrician/and maintenance man for my church, as well as periodically driving an activity bus for the school I teach at, doing jewelry repair, and renovating the house we live in. Since I was in my early twenties, I have regularly worked in the neighborhood of ninety hours per week.

And yet, as I write these words on February 18, 2025, I have not yet missed a single day of working out this year.

Let me explain how that works, because I am not trying to brag; I am trying to help people.

Let's start from the beginning; that always seems like a logical choice. And by beginning, I mean the beginning of every single day.

What do Republicans and Democrats, liberals and conservatives, men and women, black and white, capitalists and communists, and even Georgia Bulldog and Alabama Crimson Tide fans have in common?

Everyone sleeps and then gets out of bed.

Now, before I ever get out of bed in the morning, I have already done several important things every single day. When my alarm clock goes off, the first thing I do is spend some time in prayer right there in bed. The next thing I do is read my Bible. The next thing I do is post a Bible verse across all of my social media platforms. Then I post a book quote. Then I send my DO Drops daily devotional text to all of my church members.

And then my feet hit the floor. But about ten to fifteen seconds later, my back hits the floor. We have a chair in the corner of our bedroom, and I use it to start my exercise for the day with a core workout every single day. In eight to ten minutes, I have done crunches and flutter kicks and reverse crunches and planks and few other core exercises.

Every. Day.

"Well, eight to ten minutes isn't very impressive," sniffs the scoffer.

To which I say, "Thank you for proving my point." It is indeed a very tiny amount of time – meaning that pretty much everyone has time to do the exact same thing I am doing. But the cool thing is, over the course of a year, I end up doing nearly 30,000 crunches, 40,000 flutter kicks, and so on. And while only my wife will ever see me without a shirt if I can help it, you will have to trust me when I tell you that I have fairly well-defined abs and a super-strong core because of that tiny amount of time each day. And many days, I add body-weight calf raises and squats and pushups and a few other quick exercises to the mix.

Later, though, I schedule a full workout. For me, it is often mid-morning, sometimes early evening, and other times even pretty late at night. I usually work in a six-day rotation. Day one is chest, day two is biceps, day three is triceps, day four is back, day five is shoulders, and day six is legs. And while a full workout for any of those body groupings can last as long as an hour and a half if my schedule allows, any of them can also be done in thirty minutes or less if my schedule requires. So, on a really tight day, eight minutes in the morning, thirty minutes at some other point during the day, and I still have plenty of time to get everything else done.

"You make that sound so easy, but I could never even spare those thirty-eight minutes!" says Madam Excusemaker.

Are you sure?

In years past, I might have agreed with you. But then it dawned on me that every second that I spent watching television or scrolling on my phone or playing video games was time that I could put to better use. I spend very, very little time on the things that atrophy both brains and body; each rotation of the Earth around its axis goes by far too quickly for me to waste many moments.

But what of the days when everything goes haywire, and you get home very late, feeling like you have been run through a ringer?

Feel free to ask my wife how many times I have gone down into our basement gym (sometimes in a suit and tie!) to do a quick workout. See, there is a rule of exercise that I made up and have chosen to live by:

If you do not have time to do everything, just do one thing.

Chest day, but I get home at 9:45 PM? That stinks. But I am probably going down into the gym and putting a light weight (for me, maybe 135) on the bar and lifting it as many times as possible in ten minutes or so. Biceps day, and I am dragging in from a meeting? I am likely heading downstairs to grab the 30-pound curl bar and doing a couple of hundred curls really quickly.

It dawns on me that I should probably address something that you have probably already thought about (and maybe shouted at me over), namely, the fact that I keep on talking about our gym in our basement, while not everyone has one of those.

We are indeed blessed in that situation. I have a full basement of roughly 1000 square feet, and it is jam-packed with high-quality gym equipment. If you can do something like that, I highly recommend it. If you cannot, I highly recommend that you get a monthly membership to a good local gym. But even if you cannot do that either, the morning routine that I mentioned can be done by everyone, and, with a few small pieces of equipment that take up very little room, you can still do a good and thorough workout at home.

One of the best things you can get is a quality set of adjustable dumbbells. I actually have a set in my office at church, another set in my bedroom, and I use both pretty regularly. Each one can be adjusted from 10 to 50 pounds. All by themselves, they are enough for me to do an adequate biceps workout, shoulders, triceps, some leg work, and even a decent amount of chest work and back work. A good friend of mine, Chris "The Bearded Beast" Hewett (my name for him, for which I expect a heartfelt thank you when he reads this), uses resistance bands better than anyone I have ever seen. And a good set of those can fit in a tiny drawer!

Time. It is all about how to use your time. My choice has been to put exercise ahead of other things of lesser importance. I will often eat lunch at my desk to allow time for a workout later.

So don't you dare say it.

But I will say this for the third time now in this book:

You can do this!

Chapter Four
Chew on This a While

Unless you are an Olympic swimmer in your prime, the old maxim probably applies to you:

You can't out-exercise bad eating habits.

I know a few people who exercise four or five times a week. I know a very few people who exercise every single day. There are even a few utterly psychotic people (It's me; I'm the psychotic people) who often work out multiple times a day. But I do not know anyone who works out three times a day, every single day.

But just about everyone eats three meals every single day, plus snacks in between meals. So, if those meals and snacks are trying to kill you, and your workouts are trying to save you, most people have thirty-five periods of time during their week fighting against them (21 meals, 14 snack breaks) and only four or five periods of time trying to help them live. Mathematically, that simply does not work out well.

The only way that can change is to turn some of those thirty-five enemies into allies.

Better yet, you can turn nearly all of those thirty-five enemies into allies; you can make your meals work with your workouts toward your good health rather than against that goal.

I want to tell you right up front that if you are expecting this chapter to present you with some cutting-edge, complicated information that you have trouble pronouncing or remembering, you will be disappointed. People live in the real world; trying to get them to subsist on some weird combination of exotic fruits and vegetables cooked a certain way and eaten at a certain time, followed by expensive supplements that they have trouble pronouncing, let alone finding, is neither feasible nor necessary, in my opinion.

So let me just tell you what I have learned through long personal experience and a bit of my own research through the years. I will put this list in simple rule form so that you can easily remember or refer back to it.

Rule number one: don't drink bad stuff.

Your first assumption upon reading that rule is likely that I have alcohol in mind. But while I am absolutely, adamantly opposed to drinking any alcohol at all, both for moral and for health reasons, that is only one thing I have in mind here, and not even the main thing.

The main things I have in mind are sugar, calories, chemicals, and carbonation.

I have pretty much lost count of all the people I have known who exercised really hard and yet verbally bemoaned their inability to lose weight and get fit in between big slurps of their Sundrop, Mountain Dew, and sugar with a bit of tea mixed in. In case you have not bothered to run the numbers, a 20-ounce Sundrop has 290 calories, a 20-ounce Mountain Dew has 280 calories, and a typical glass of sweet tea at a restaurant has 200 calories. And making that last one all the worse for my dear friends here in the South, you probably have that tea glass refilled at least twice while you are at the table, and then get a to-go cup for the road. It is not uncommon for 800-1000 calories to slide down the gullet of any normal tea drinker at every single meal!

Let me put that in southern sciencey terms:

That's turrible.

Kool-Aid? Yeah, same.

"But fruit juices are okay, because they're from fruit, right?"

Please don't give me a migraine. The occasional glass of squeezed orange juice is a good thing, unsweetened grapefruit juice is better, but most fruit juices are loaded with their own natural sugar plus extra sugar to satisfy the American sweet tooth. And the calorie content is high either way.

"Hah! I'm good; I'm a coffee drinker!"

Are you? Are you really? Or are you a sugary creamer drinker with a hint of coffee added in?

Again, the occasional coffee with creamer is not going to kill you. But if your drink of choice throughout the day is coffee loaded with sugary, high-calorie creamer, you can run on your treadmill until it runs away from home, and you are not likely to make any progress on weight loss or fitness goals. The average person in America could change their life dramatically just by changing what they drink; what could be easier than that?

When Dana and I got married, water was a curse word to me, tea had to have enough sugar in it to make a spoon stand up straight, coffee was mixed with creamer and caramel and whipped cream and served over ice, and Coca-Cola was a multiple times a day experience. And in spite of how hard I worked and/or worked out, my weight started to rise (along with my blood pressure), and I was not breathing well.

Instinctively, I started eyeballing my beverages.

I did not know much, but I figured that maybe I would start with "less bad" versions of my favorites. I started drinking diet sodas and tea sweetened with artificial sweeteners. The result? I lost a couple of pounds, the breathing did not improve at all, and I started having splitting headaches.

Instinctively, I started eyeballing my beverages yet again.

Could I do it? Could I really lay aside those lifelong comfort drinks?

I made up my mind to try. I started with cutting out all soft drinks, and thus all carbonation; I strictly drank tea sweetened with artificial sweeteners. My breathing got markedly better – and my headaches stayed as bad as ever.

No, please, not that...

I started eyeballing my beverages yet again. Was it even possible? Could a southern-born and bred North Carolinian really do it?

I switched to unsweetened tea and started drinking water copiously as well. Everything changed; headaches are now very rare, I breathe wonderfully, and I have no trouble staying at my desired weight. I still drink the occasional milk or glass of orange/grapefruit juice or cup of coffee, but ninety-five percent of every drop of liquid that goes in my mouth is water or unsweet tea. And as a cool and unexpected benefit, I can now actually taste the tea I am drinking. I often steep mine with mint I have grown in my garden, and I can taste the mint as well.

Water is your friend. Tea (cold or hot) is your friend. Coffee minus the sugar is your friend. Milk and orange/grapefruit juice (along with other pure fruit juices) in moderation are your friends. Most other liquids are trying to kill you through heart disease, cancer, or other awful means and should either be avoided altogether or at least enjoyed only in careful moderation.

Rule number two: avoid Frankenfood.

Let me ask you about a sound; are you very familiar with how cellophane sounds as it is ripped open?

If so, you are probably eating a bunch of Frankenfood.

I obviously draw this term Frankenfood from Mary Shelly's fictional Frankenstein, an ugly, cobbled assembly of dead things that should never have been mashed together. There was nothing natural about Frankenstein, and the result was monstrous.

Just like most of what passes for food in America.

Consider the contrast between the lowly home-made pot roast and a staple of the American diet, the standard, big-box store, popular company that shall remain nameless, Oatmeal Cream Pie.

The standard pot roast has water, beef, onions, carrots, celery, garlic, potatoes, brown sugar, salt, and pepper.

The Oatmeal Cream Pie has "a few" more and more complicated ingredients. Specifically, one of those admittedly delectable treats is made of oats, fructose, molasses, dextrose, degerminated yellow corn meal, soybean oil, palm oil, non-fat milk, whey, soy lecithin, vanilla, unspecified artificial and natural flavors, caramel color, cinnamon, nutmeg, baking soda, baking powder, raisin paste, chocolate, cocoa, yellow dye number five, red dye number forty, yellow dye number six, and blue dye number one.

I am not singling out one food item from one company, here: I am pointing to a larger trend and a comparison between mostly natural and largely unnatural. Try this: go through the supermarket sometime and read the labels on prepackaged foods and snacks. You are going to find a startling percentage of our food supply that has monstrous numbers of ingredients, many of which you cannot pronounce or identify.

Now, if, by chance, Frankenfoods were healthier and lower in calories than natural foods, they may be a good idea. But as far as I can tell, that is rarely the case. In addition to containing things that I do not want in my system, that Oatmeal Cream Pie has 170 calories, or 490 for the double-decker!

A banana comes in at 105 calories, and wants to help you.

Processed meats are a culprit here as well. I used to think that all meat was protein, and thus a good option. But then one day it dawned on me that "meat" doesn't come in those perfect tube or can shapes. What does come in them is meat and other particles that have been mashed and mangled together, generally with binding agents to hold it all together. Per the World Health Organization, processed meats increase the risk of certain cancers, are linked to cardiovascular disease, contribute to type 2 diabetes, contain nitrates and nitrites (Hint: those are generally pretty bad for you), and are high in saturated fat.

Am I occasionally going to eat some packaged treat or meat? Occasionally, yes. Rarely, but occasionally. But the vast majority of the time, I am going to eat fruits, vegetables, good proteins (eggs, meat, some cheese, etc.) quality carbs (baked potatoes, sweet potatoes, rice, whole wheat or sourdough bread in moderation, etc.) and other natural foods that come from the ground or from a tree or from nature with no stop at a Frankenfactory before it gets to my table.

Rule number three: don't fry/don't die.

We are Americans, or 'Muricans, amiright? As such, we fry our chicken, okra (oakree, for my fellow southerners), taters, squash (skwarsh), onions, pork chops, tomatoes, catfish, shrimp, and, I kid you not, even our Oreos and ice cream. If you think I am making those last two up, go visit any county fair and then get back to me.

But to put it mildly, that is a bad choice compared to other methods of food preparation. Mind you, just like with everything else we have discussed thus far, the occasional treat is not likely to kill you. A Cajun fillet biscuit here or there is not the real issue for most; the real issue is that, as a whole, frying/deep frying foods pack on a ton of calories and a ton of potential harm for the heart and arteries. A grilled, five-ounce chicken breast is going to have around 210 calories, while that same five-ounce chicken breast will have 381 calories when fried. You are nearly doubling the calories just by the preparation method!

Let me explain in plain and approximate terms what this means. You are sitting at a table with your entire day of food in front of you. Your friend is sitting across from you with that exact same setup of food, item for item. But while your neighbor has one hundred percent grilled, baked, or broiled food, fifty percent of your food has been fried.

Congratulations; with the exact same amount of food on your plate as on his, you now have 4,500 calories to his 3,000 calories, and his food is not actively trying to clog his arteries.

Rule number four: don't overeat.

Why, oh why is this even necessary to explain? But trust me, it is indeed necessary.

Many years ago, my father-in-law sat down to eat with a well-known preacher. He was large; very large. When the waitress came to the table to take their order, the preacher said, "I'll have a pound of bacon and a dozen eggs; I'll start with that."

She laughed – and then choked back her laughter when she realized that he was absolutely serious. And he was; she brought him a pound of bacon and a dozen eggs, he polished all of it off, and then started in on the pancakes.

And he also died fairly young; he dug his own grave with a spoon. A man who was being mightily used of God drastically cut short his service, along with his life.

At this point, you may be expecting me to delve into a discussion of how many calories a day you will need to take in based on your height, weight, gender, and age. But I will not do that for one simple reason: absolutely everyone is different in ways that significantly impact caloric needs. Some have a very high metabolism, some much lower. Some are very active all during the day, others sit at a desk. Some work out hard and regularly, others are more sporadic.

With all the differences and variables, trying to come up with a proper number of calories for everyone is a fool's errand.

So, how are you supposed to know if you are overeating or not?

Here is a simple template.

One: If you are gorging yourself, you are taking in too many calories. This should not be too hard for you or those you love to recognize.

Two: If you feel bloated or miserable after eating a meal, you are taking in too many calories.

Three: If you are gaining (non-muscle) weight and there is no medical issue causing that weight gain, you are almost certainly taking in too many calories.

Four: If you are healthy and regularly exercising and not losing weight while trying to do so, you are probably taking in too many calories.

Five: If you are healthy and fit and maintaining the weight you have, you are likely taking in the right amount of calories

Six: If you are trying to lose weight and are successfully pulling off a little bit of weight each week, you are likely taking in the right amount of calories for what you are trying to do.

Seven: If you are not morbidly obese, and are trying to lose weight, and are losing a large amount of weight in a very short period of time, you are probably taking in too few calories to maintain health, strength, and bone density while you lose weight.

Eight: If you are working out and trying to gain muscle mass, yet staying at the same weight, you are probably taking in too few calories, and need to eat some extra portions of lean protein and high-quality carbs.

In a way, it is as much artwork as science. You are your own unique masterpiece, a creation of God, a one-of-a-kind that will never be repeated. The life you live is just as unique. Therefore, you will want to tweak and adjust your personal eating habits until you start achieving your personal goals.

A few years ago, when I was lifting extremely heavy, I intentionally bulked up to right at 212 pounds. Honestly, that was a bit heavy for my five-foot nine-and-a-half inches, but it did allow me a personal best of 355 on the bench press. But when I started feeling miserable and my knees started hurting, I decided to pull some of that weight off. I now range between 190 and 195 pounds of really solid muscle. That is a decrease in body weight of 22 pounds or so. And I did not do it by counting calories; I did it by eating a bit less volume each day, and by eating things that I knew were a bit lower in caloric content. And when the weight started dropping a pound or two each week, I knew I had hit the sweet spot. I then kept eating roughly that amount and type until I reached my goal, and then adjusted to simply maintain where I was at.

I step on the scale pretty much every morning; if it is in my desired range, I go about my day of eating as normal. If it has crept up a bit beyond that, I back my volume of food down for the day, or eat things like salads and veggies and avoid breads. The next day, it will be back in range.

"But I will always be hungry!"

No, you won't, not if you learn to eat things that are both filling and lower in calories than other foods. Instead of breads and sweets, fill up on vegetables (a cup of cooked broccoli is filling, yet contains only 55 calories!) fruits (1 apple, just 95 calories) legumes, whole grains, lean proteins, broth-based soups (1 cup of vegetable soup, 100 calories) air popped pop corn (3 cups, just 90 calories) Greek yogurt (a six ounce serving, just 100 calories) cottage cheese (half a cup of 1% fat just 80 calories) and mushrooms (1 cup of cooked mushrooms, just 40 calories).

There are many more you can find. Look for foods that are high in water content, fiber, and protein. Go find the foods that make you feel full, but do so on comparatively few calories.

Fitness and health almost always start with what you put in your mouth.

You. Can. Do. This!

Section 2
Let's Workout!

Chapter Five
An Overview

When it comes to working out, the first thing you should know is that I am right and everyone else is wrong, and that I have finally figured it all out after centuries of people floundering in darkness and ignorance on the subject. I know this because *that is how nearly every fitness guy/girl everywhere portrays things!*

The two problems are, one, it is never true, and two, it shows a monstrous lack of humility that always makes me want to say, "Dude, back off on the 'roids long enough to not be a donkey for just a bit."

I work out, and I think I do it pretty well. But there are a lot of other really, really good guys and girls out there giving really good advice as well, things born out of years of their own experiences. So if you are able to benefit from what I teach you here, wonderful. If you find help elsewhere, still wonderful. If you figure out on your own what works best for you, yep, still wonderful.

So I am going to teach you what I know and how I do it. I am also going to tap some other solid people on subjects that they know better than I do, and allow them to help you here in this book.

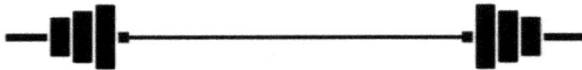

I am a powerlifter. That is a distinction I want to make, since I often get called a bodybuilder. Those two things are often somewhat similar, but they do have some real differences. For starters, I will never be on a stage posing for people; as a Christian, I understand that most of my body is only for my wife's viewing pleasure. Secondly, powerlifters are primarily concerned with being able to lift heavy things, hence the compound word power-lifting.

That said, there is a general term that encompasses both of those things pretty well, and that is the generic term weight lifter. And that is a good term for us to remember, since a lot of what I am going to teach you in this section of the book is how to lift weights.

But weightlifting is not all there is to working out and to fitness. In fact, one of the things that is the very best for fitness is something that I hopefully do not need to teach anyone, namely, walking!

Wouldn't that make for a fun video: "Here we go, ladies and gentlemen, I am going to extend my left leg until the heel makes light contact with the ground. Then I am going to shift my weight forward a bit until the ball of the foot also makes contact with the ground. At this point, if you will watch carefully, I am going to transfer my weight to the right side of my body, shift forward a bit on that side, and let my right heel make contact with the ground. As it does, you will notice that my left heel has begun to leave the ground, and I am up on the ball of my left foot. I will now lift that left foot off of the ground at the same time that the ball of my right foot makes contact with the ground, and then we will repeat the entire process again for the next step..."

Yeah, I am pretty sure I don't need to do a video on that, or on swimming, or on jogging.

But while I will do no video on those, we will discuss those kinds of things in general. The point is not to get you to do every little thing I do; the point is to get you fit and strong and healthy.

So here is the plan. For the next several chapters, I am going to tell you how I work out, describe the exercises in detail, group them by muscle groups, and even provide pictures and videos.

Hey, you! You can do this!

Chapter Six
My Six-Day Routine

When you talk to different people who work out, you will quickly find that they are *different people*. Some primarily do full body workouts whenever they work out, very briefly hitting every single muscle group and then moving on to the next. Others major on one particular muscle group (usually chest or legs) and do that nearly every day, while sprinkling other muscle group workouts in periodically. Others mix push or pull muscle groups (for example, back and biceps, chest and shoulders) and thus hit them multiple times a week. I separate muscle groups six distinct ways: chest, biceps, triceps, back, shoulders, legs (remember, I do core every morning).

So, which way is correct?

Mine, of course; everyone else is an incompetent loser.

I'm very obviously kidding. The actual answer is, any of those methodologies is fine and dandy. But since my way has worked for me, I am going to teach you my way. If you choose to do it in a different way, have at it; just *do it.*

That list of groups I gave you above is not just the six ways I divide the muscle groupings; it is also the order in which I work them. I work chest, then the next day I work biceps, then the next day I work triceps, then the next day I work back, then the next day I work shoulders, then the next day I work legs, then I start over with chest.

Here is the method behind my madness. Chest exercises are primarily pushing exercises: bench press, pushups, dumbbell presses, etc. So the next day, I want to do primarily pulling exercises, hence, biceps day. The next day, I want to push again, and triceps are mostly pushing exercises. Then comes back day, which is mostly pulling, followed by shoulders, which is mostly pushing. And then comes legs. And while legs are mostly pushing, every other day has been upper body, so the legs are rested and ready.

By using that methodology, my muscles get two of the three things they need to grow and thrive: exercise and rest (the third, of course, is proper nutrients). When I do chest, most everything but the chest is getting some rest (I say "most" because there is always some bleed over; most chest exercises also somewhat hit the triceps and shoulders, for instance). When I do biceps, most everything else is getting rest, though the back is engaged a bit on most biceps exercises.

You get the point. By separating the muscle groups, I can work out day after day after day and still have my muscle groups get most of the rest they need to grow and thrive. And this day after day system is also beneficial for those seeking to lose weight, since you burn calories every time you work out.

Not every workout I do is the same. If you want to make progress, you need to remember this scientific maxim:

Sameness is lameness.

Yes, I made that up; please, no applause, just throw high-quality weight gloves my way.

Here is what I mean by sameness is lameness. Your muscles are, like the rest of you, stubborn. They want more than anything to get into a comfortable groove and *then be left alone.* And when they get into that comfortable groove, that routine rut, they will stagnate. The way to avoid that bad outcome is to change things up from time to time to keep challenging those muscles.

Let's take bench press as an example, since I like it more than anything else. In case you didn't know, in heaven, every day is chest day (I hope).

My normal routine is to warm up with light weight (20 reps of the 45lb bar, then 10 reps of 135 lbs) and then move up in weight pretty quickly. I will normally jump straight to 2 reps of 225, then one rep of 275, and then will max out at somewhere around 315-335 pounds. I will then drop back to 275 for 2 or 3 reps, then drop in weight by ten pounds each remaining set, doing as many reps as possible all the way back down to 225, which I will normally rep fifteen times or so by that point.

After a few weeks of that, though, I switch gears. I will start at 135, then add ten pounds of weight each set, doing reps of ten until I cannot get to ten reps. Normally, somewhere around 245, I will find that I can only do seven or eight. Then I will keep adding ten pounds, doing as many reps as possible, which decreases each time. By about 285 pounds, I will be gassed and only able to do one rep. I will then keep trying ten pounds heavier (with a spotter) until I fail.

The next day, my chest will let me know that it is not happy with me, but that the workout was worth the effort.

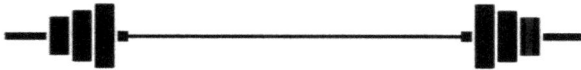

Now that you know that things need to be changed up periodically, let me give you my entire, standard six-day workout routine. Here goes.

Day One: Chest

Flat bench press, from lighter to max, then back to a lower yet still reasonably heavy weight. For me, this usually works out to eleven sets or so. (You will find that my first exercise every day gets a ton of sets and reps, and everything following gets three sets.)

The flat bench press is a fantastic exercise for building the front and center of the chest. If you only have time for one angle of bench press each day, make it the standard flat bench press. It will hit a bigger portion of the chest than any of the other angles.

Incline bench press, three sets. The incline bench press is a fantastic exercise for the upper bands of the chest and also incorporates the shoulders and triceps. Since I have already warmed up on the standard flat bench press, I will start with my heaviest weight on this, a weight that I know I can get 4-6 reps of. Then I will drop in weight each of the next two sets, using a weight that I can get 8 to 10 reps of. For me, this is usually 225, 205, 185.

Decline bench press, three sets. The decline bench press is a fantastic exercise for the lower bands of the chest, and also heavily incorporates both the shoulders and triceps into the movement. It has a reduced range of motion from the other two types of bench press, and most people can lift more on the decline bench press than on any other angle of bench press. I will start with my heaviest weight on this, a weight that I know I can get 4 to 6 reps of. Then I will drop in weight each of the next two sets, using a weight that I can get 8 to 10 reps of. For me, by this point in the workout, this is usually 275, 245, 225.

Dumbbell press, three sets. The dumbbell bench press is a fantastic exercise for the chest, and also heavily incorporates the shoulders and triceps and even the abdominal muscles. It also engages stabilizer muscles in the core and back. I will start with my heaviest weight on this, a weight that I know I can get 10-12 reps of. Then I will drop in weight each of the next two sets, using a weight that I can still get 8 to 10 reps of. For me, by this point in the workout, this is usually a set of 100-pounders, then 90s, then 80s.

Dumbbell center press, three sets (also called Crush Press). The dumbbell center press is a great exercise for the very center of the chest; if you want definition in your chest, this is an exercise you will want to incorporate. I will start with my heaviest weight on this, a weight that I know I can get 15-17 reps of. Then I will drop in weight each of the next two sets, using a weight that

I can still get 12-15 reps of. For me, by this point in the workout, this is usually a set of 50-pounders, then 40s, then 30s.

Cable flies, three sets. The cable fly is a great exercise for definition in the chest and is also very joint-friendly. I generally keep the weight the same for each of my three sets on this, utilizing a weight that I can get 12 to 15 reps each time.

Pushups, as many as possible, one set. This is an old gym staple, and for good reason. It may well be the most beneficial exercise for the chest that mankind has available, in spite of modern equipment.

Day two: Biceps

Close-grip chin-ups. This is an excellent exercise for the biceps, the back, and also for the brachialis, which is somewhat beneath the biceps itself, and when worked, helps to give the biceps a bigger appearance. I will start with an assisted chin-up machine, drop in counterweight until I do pure body weight chin-ups, then do a set of weighted chin-ups, then a finishing set of several assisted chin-ups. This normally works out to about ten or eleven sets for me, and at the heaviest point, I will be doing body weight plus a 31-pound chain draped over my shoulders.

Hammer curl chin-ups, three sets, body weight. This is an excellent exercise for the peak of the biceps, also known as the long head. If you want your biceps to appear taller, not just wider, any hammer movement is a good option.

Barbell curls, three sets. This is another great exercise for the biceps. I will use a comparatively low weight on this and utilize it for all three sets. I want something that I can rep 10-12 times on the first set, then 8-10 times on the second, then 6-8 on the third.

Reverse cable curls, three sets. This exercise, in addition to engaging the biceps, also heavily engages the forearms, making it a truly useful exercise. It can be done with dumbbells, a barbell, or a cable and handle. I prefer the cable, because it keeps constant tension throughout the movement. I utilize a weight that I can do 12-15 reps of on the first set, 10-12 on the second, and 8-10 on the third.

Wrist curls, three sets. This is another helpful exercise for the forearms and greatly improves overall grip strength as well. I use the barbell for this, and a decreasing weight on the three sets. For me, this will normally be 25 reps of 65 pounds, 25 reps of 55 pounds, and 25 reps of 45 pounds. It may not sound like much, but the idea of this is to really focus on the wrist and forearms to the exclusion of all other muscles.

Dumbbell hammer curls, three sets. This is an excellent exercise for the peak of the biceps. I will utilize decreasing weight for each set, using a weight that I can do 15-17 reps on for the first set, 12-15 on the second, and 10-12 on the last.

Easy Bar Curl, three sets. I like this as a finishing exercise on biceps day – or as a stand-alone exercise on any day that I am rushed and can only do one thing. It is excellent for the entire biceps. As a finishing exercise, I will utilize the same weight for three reps, and do as many as I can possibly do in each set, utilizing a controlled, non-swaying motion.

Day three: Triceps

Dips. This is one of my very favorite exercises, and the one that I believe to be the most helpful both for overall power and for functionality. It helps to build the triceps, but also the chest and shoulders. It can also help you break plateaus on your bench press. I will start with the assisted dip machine, do several sets with decreasing assisted weight, then do a set of pure body weight, then several increasing sets of weighted dips, followed by a finishing set of as many body weight dips as possible. In a normal workout, this has me going as high as using two forty-five-pound plates around my waist for 6-7 reps.

On that bit about it helping to break a bench press plateau, please understand that this is not for general fitness. If you happen to be one of those individuals, though, who are trying to lift very heavy weights on the bench press and have found yourself stuck, I have found that laying off the bench press for a while and focusing on doing very heavy weighted dips tends to help me break the plateau when I go back to the bench press.

Close-grip bench press, three sets. This is a tremendous exercise to increase size and power in the triceps. I normally do three sets, decreasing in weight each time. For me, this is normally 4-6 reps of 225, 6-8 reps of 205, and 8-10 reps of 185.

Rope pulls, three sets. This is an isolation exercise that helps to both grow and give definition to the triceps. I normally do three sets, decreasing in weight each time, utilizing a weight that I can get *15 to 17 reps of on the first set, 12 to 15 on the second, and 12 or so on the third.

About that asterisk... Those reps are standard "spread reps," reps where I pull the rope down and spread it at the bottom. The reason I asterisk that is because I go on to finish with a flurry of several more reps with my hands tight together.

Bar push down, three sets. This is another great exercise for the triceps. You can use either a straight bar or an easy bar for this exercise; I generally choose the easy bar. I normally keep the same weight for all three sets, something that I can do 15 to 17 reps on the first set, 12 to 15 on the second, and 12 or so on the third.

Well pumps, three sets. Full disclosure, here: I have never actually seen anybody else do this exercise, so the name I have given it is my own. Nonetheless, I personally have found it to be one of the best exercises for giving a good burn to the triceps. I do three sets of fairly heavy decreasing weight on these, something that I can do 15 to 17 reps on the first set, 12 to 15 on the second, and 12 or so on the third.

Reverse triceps curls, three sets. This is a fantastic exercise for overall triceps development. I will keep the weight the same for all three sets, and utilize a weight that I can get twelve or so reps of each time.

Overhead rope pulls, three sets. This is a variation of the behind-the-head dumbbell press. I like it better, mostly because it is much easier on the shoulders, with much less risk of injury to said shoulders. It also keeps consistent tension throughout the motion. I will do three sets of the weight that I can do 12 or so reps of. For me, that is generally 100 to 110 pounds, though it can vary from machine to machine.

Day four: Back

Wide grip pull-ups. This is a phenomenal exercise for the lats and helps to produce the V shape in the back. I will start on the assisted machine, doing several sets that gradually decrease in assistance, then do a set of pure body weight, then a set lightly weighted, then a finishing set of lightly assisted.

Stiff-legged dead lifts, light weight, three sets. This is a very underutilized exercise in most gyms – and that is a shame, because it is an incredibly beneficial exercise, and works multiple important muscles. It helps to give strength to the lower back and produces explosive power in the hamstrings as well. It should be done with relatively light weight; form means everything in this exercise. I normally do three sets of 135, 12 reps in each. Even if all you use is the 45-pound bar or a set of dumbbells, though, this is still a great and beneficial exercise.

Lat pull-downs, three sets. Similar to the wide grip pull-up, this targets the lats and helps to produce a wide, strong, V-shaped back. I generally do three sets of the weight that I can do 12 or so reps of, and I go reasonably heavy on this, but not so heavy that I jerk the bar and cable. A smooth, steady motion, both down and up, is what you want on this.

Narrow grip lat pull downs, three sets. This still targets the back, but also hits the biceps pretty hard as well; a lot of back exercises incorporate the biceps. The only difference is the grip width; I still do three sets of reasonably heavy weight, something that I can get around 12 reps of each time.

Stiff arm bar push down, three sets. This targets the lats – provided you do it correctly. As a nice bonus, it also hits the front of the shoulders pretty well. I generally do three sets of the weight that I can do 12 or so reps of, and once again, a smooth, steady motion, both down and up, is what you want on this.

Low row, three sets. This exercise is an underutilized gem that targets more muscle groups than most. It will primarily benefit your back, specifically the lats, rhomboids, and trapezius muscles, but will also benefit your rear delts, biceps, erector spinae (spine muscles), and even your calves and, *ahem,* your backside. You can do this using a specific low row machine, or you can use a cable machine and many different widths of handle attachments (I prefer the Double D row handle). I do three sets of this, using decently heavy weight, but slow, controlled movements both in and back. I aim for 12-15 reps with each set.

Dante row, three sets. The Dante row is not as well-known as many other exercises for the back, but it is genuinely one of the best. It isolates and activates the lats as good or better than anything else you can do. I do three sets of the same weight, decently heavy, and aim for 10-12 reps with each set.

Bar twist, one set. This very effectively activates the stabilizer muscles. It is the last thing I do on back day, so I do one set from each side, generally aiming for 12-15 reps each way.

You will notice I did not include the standard deadlift. It can be a fantastic exercise – it can also do a lot of damage to a back, so I do not do it very often. I will show you how to do it, courtesy of my fantastic (and super strong) Assistant Pastor, Brandon Tolley, but I personally am very sparing with it and have managed to build an extremely strong back without it.

Here is the link to that video:

Day five: Shoulders

Behind-the-head shoulder press, several sets, not too heavy. This is a fantastic exercise – but also a damaging one if done improperly or too heavily. It engages the entire shoulder, but in particular the rear delts. If you already have damaged shoulders, do not do this exercise. If you have healthy shoulders and the discipline to do the exercise properly and with a sensible weight, it is incredibly beneficial.

I do several sets of this, starting with just the 45-pound bar itself for 20 reps. Then I move up ten pounds each set, doing reps of 10 until that is too much, then doing a couple more sets of lower reps. I normally go no higher than 135 pounds, and often even stop as low as 95 pounds.

Machine shoulder press, three sets. This is a great and generally safe way to work the shoulders, and most every gym has one. I generally do three sets of decreasing weight, and aim for 10-12 reps each time.

Shoulder shrug, three sets. These are mainly for the traps, but also work the neck to a lesser degree. If you want tall, rounded traps, these are a staple. You can do them using a barbell, dumbbells, plates, or even certain bench press machines. I generally do a minimum of three sets, and with decently heavy weight, aiming for around 20 reps per set.

Front upward push, three sets. This requires something like a standing calf machine, and it is excellent for safe shoulder development. The narrow grip hits the shoulders in a different way than most other shoulder exercises. I normally aim for three sets of 18-20 reps, which for me is 140-160 pounds.

Upright barbell row, three sets. This awkward-looking exercise is a workhorse; it activates the lateral delts, upper traps, biceps, forearms, and improves grip strength. You do not need heavy weights for this; good form is the key to getting the most out of it, not how much weight you move. I normally do three sets of somewhere around 65 pounds, and aim for 12-15 reps each set.

Crazy eights, one set. This is my own exercise; I developed it to hit the three shoulder heads from every possible angle. I use very light weight by this point in the workout – normally 10-12 pound dumbbells for this. It is eight reps to the front, eight reps at a 45-degree angle, and eight reps to the sides.

Plate shrugs, 1 set. Simply shrug a plate (I use a 45 on each side) as many times as possible.

Day six: Legs

Leg press, several sets, increasing in weight with each set, then reversing. I utilize this as my primary leg exercise rather than squats. It delivers much the same benefit as squats, while keeping the back much safer. I begin with a low weight (180 in plates, not counting the carriage), then work my way up in 90-pound increments, decreasing in reps for each set, until I do a max for one or two reps. Then I work my way back down by 90-pound increments, stopping with a set of 360 pounds, as many as I can do.

Calf press on the leg press machine, six sets. This is a great exercise for the calves, and once again has the benefit of added safety over certain forms of standing calf exercises. With the weight already where I stopped in the last exercise, I do as many calf raises as I can (usually around 30), wait fifteen seconds, then do a second set of that weight, as many reps as I can (usually 12-15). Then I will lower the weight by 90 pounds and do the same thing, then lower it again by 90 pounds and do the same thing.

Hack squat, three sets. This is another great and much safer variant of the traditional squat. With the weight already where I left off in the last exercise, I will switch the leg press to hack squat formation (if yours does not do this, you can just go to a dedicated hack squat machine) and do three sets of 10-12 reps.

Standing (or seated) calf machine, three sets. You will notice that I bounce back and forth between upper leg muscles and lower leg muscles in this routine. This gives each set a chance to rest a bit, increasing the safety. I have and use the standing calf machine, though a seated calf machine works well also. I keep the weight the same for all three sets, something that I can do 16-18 reps of.

Leg extension, three sets. This isolation exercise will give you a better burn in your quadriceps muscles (the big muscles in the front of the legs) than most any other exercise. I start with a higher weight, then decrease the weight each set, aiming for 12-15 reps each time. Some days, I do nothing but this exercise and do a great many sets of it.

Leg curls, three sets. I loathe and detest this exercise – but I do it anyway, because it is a good exercise. It is an isolation exercise that very effectively targets the hamstrings. There are machines that allow you to do it from a seated position, but most require you to lie face down. I generally do 1-3 sets, aiming for 8-10 reps each time.

You will notice that I did not include the standard barbell squat. As with the deadlift, it can be a fantastic exercise – it can also do a lot of damage to the back, so I do not do it very often. I will show you how to do it, courtesy of my fantastic (as super strong) Assistant Pastor, Brandon Tolley, but I personally am very sparing with it and have built very strong legs wthout it.

Here is the link to that squat video.

So that is my standard routine. Mind you, there are a bunch of other exercises I will sprinkle in along the way, though, just for fun and variety.

And now, let's get down to brass tacks – or more properly, steel plates.

Chapter Seven
Your Visual Guide to the Exercises

Chest

Bench Press

As you lie down on the bench, you should position yourself to where the bar is comfortable and safe for you to lift; mine will be roughly over the top of my pecs. Position your hands roughly shoulder-width apart, or just a slight bit wider. If you go too wide, you will be hitting mostly the front of your shoulders; too narrow, and you will be mostly hitting your triceps.

Keep your butt on the bench throughout the lift; so help me, if I find out you are levitating your patootie, I will commission a sniper to shoot it with a tranquilizer dart as you do. We will then send you to a re-education camp for gym Communists until you agree to do it right.

Lift the bar off the bench (have a spotter help you with a liftoff on any heavy lifts), then in a controlled manner, lower it to your solar plexus (the softy spot right below your pecs in the center of your chest) and then lift it back into place.

*Note: an advanced technique for heavier lifts is to use leg drive, pushing with your legs as if you are trying to push your body in the direction of your head. For general fitness, you do not really need to know or practice this, but for advanced lifting, it can be pretty helpful.

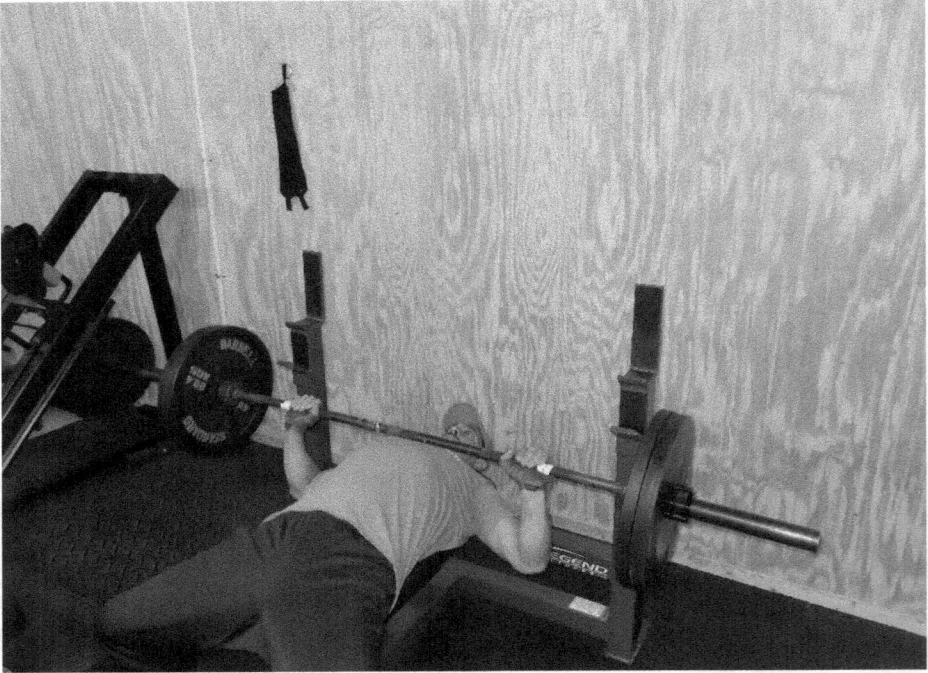

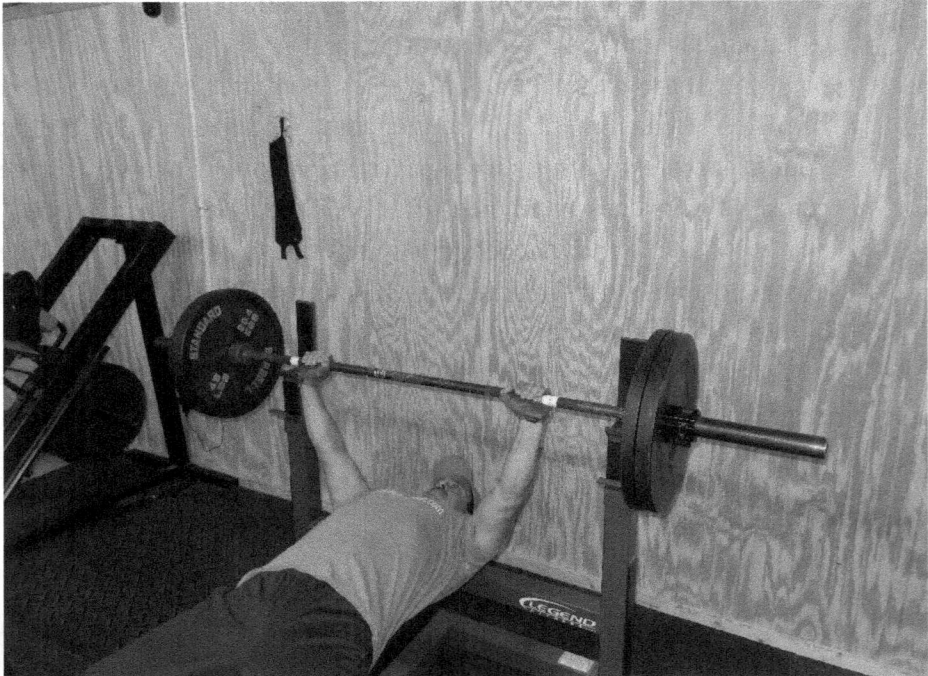

Incline bench press

As you lie back on the bench, you should position yourself to where the bar is comfortable and safe for you to lift; mine will be roughly over my chin or neck, depending on the angle of the bench. Position your hands roughly shoulder-width apart, or just a slight bit wider. Lift the bar off the bench (have a spotter help you with a liftoff on any heavy lifts), then in a controlled manner, lower it to your pecs, and then lift it back into place.

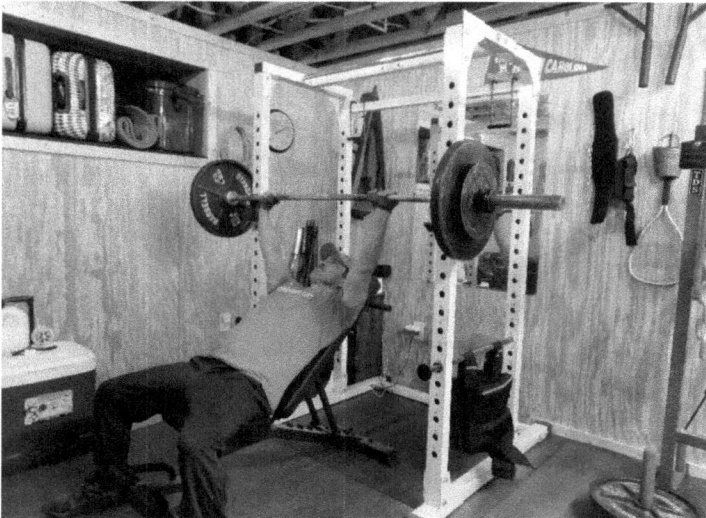

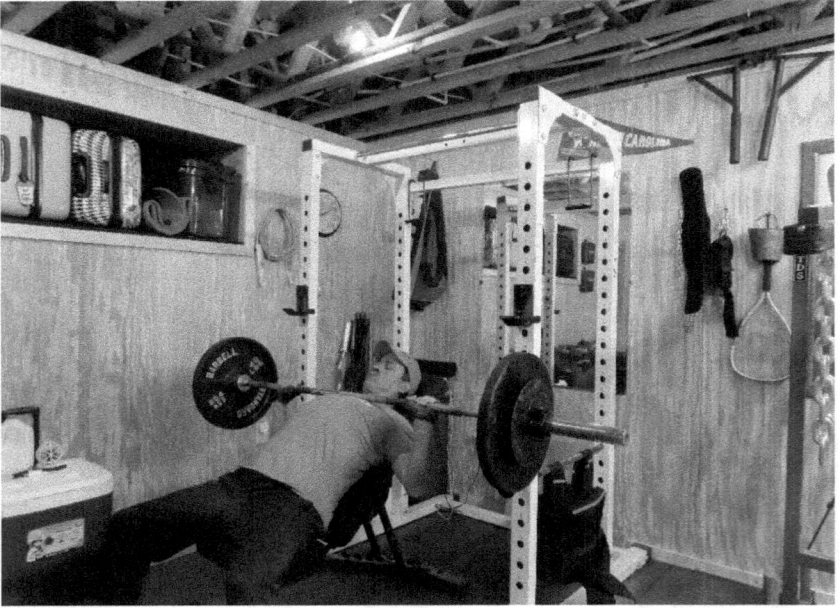

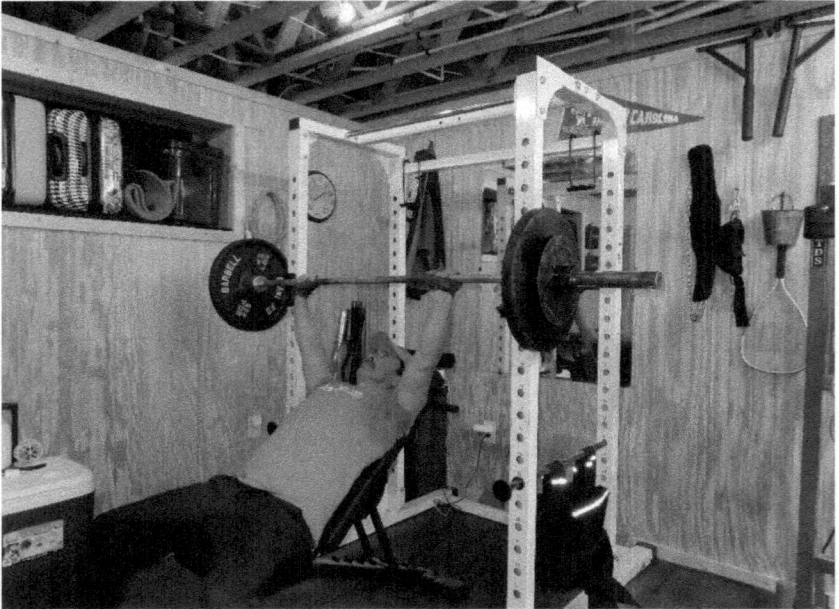

Decline bench press

As you lie back on the bench, you should position yourself to where the bar is comfortable and safe for you to lift; mine will be roughly over my high upper chest. Position your hands roughly shoulder-width apart, or just a slight bit wider. Lift the bar off the bench (have a spotter help you with a liftoff on any heavy lifts), then, in a controlled manner, lower it to the top of your stomach, and then lift it back into place.

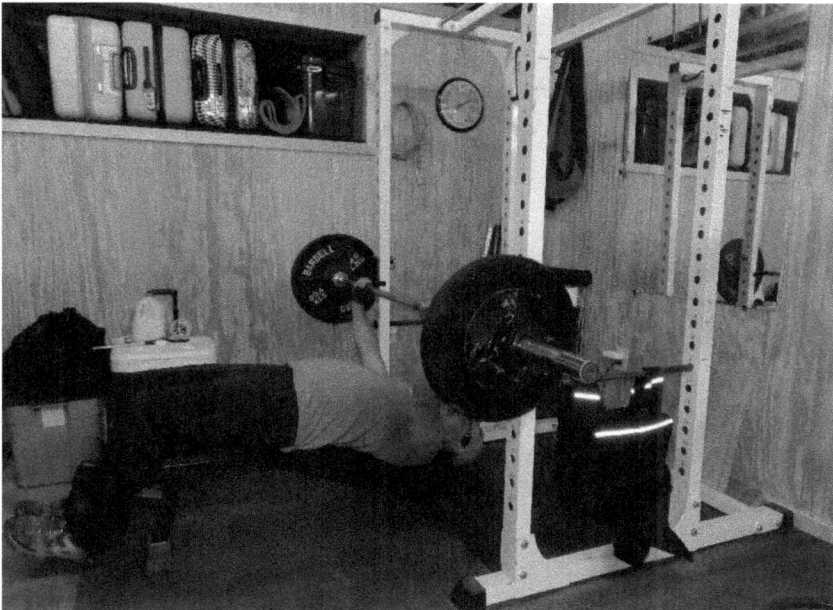

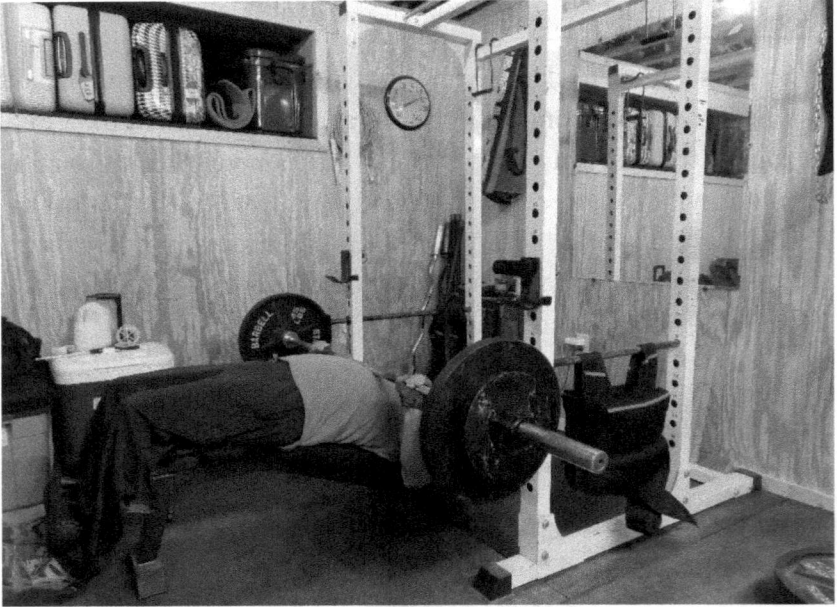

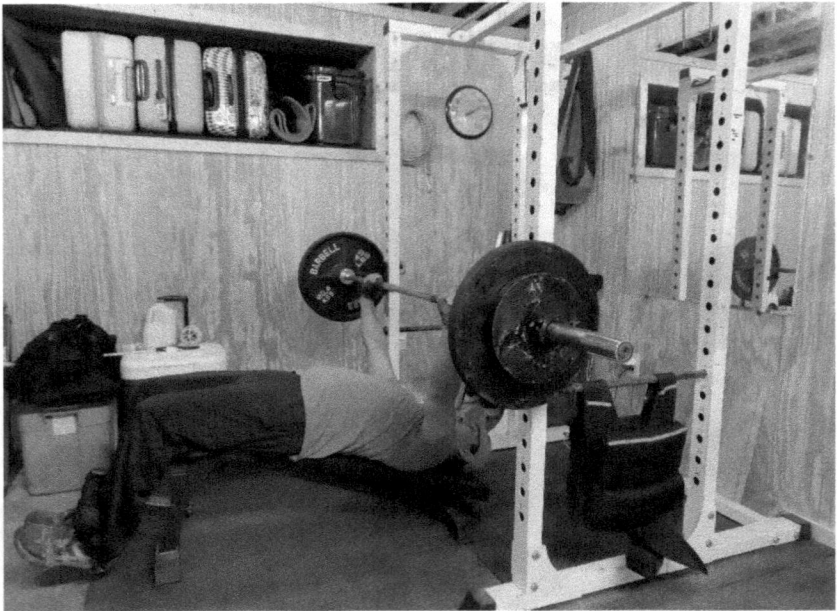

Dumbbell press

Starting from a seated position on the bench, with a dumbbell in each hand resting on each knee, lie backwards and position each dumbbell in roughly the same place as if it were the barbell in a bench press. It is helpful to turn your hands slightly outward, as if twisting your pinkies toward your feet. Bring both weights upward, over the chest, not over your face. They can come slightly inward toward each other, but do not let them make contact with each other.

Lower back down to the starting position.

When you are finished with each set, either rock your legs and body to sit up with the weights, or have someone take them from you. If you must drop them, make sure you are using rubber-coated weights and dropping them on a rubber mat, and do so as gently as possible.

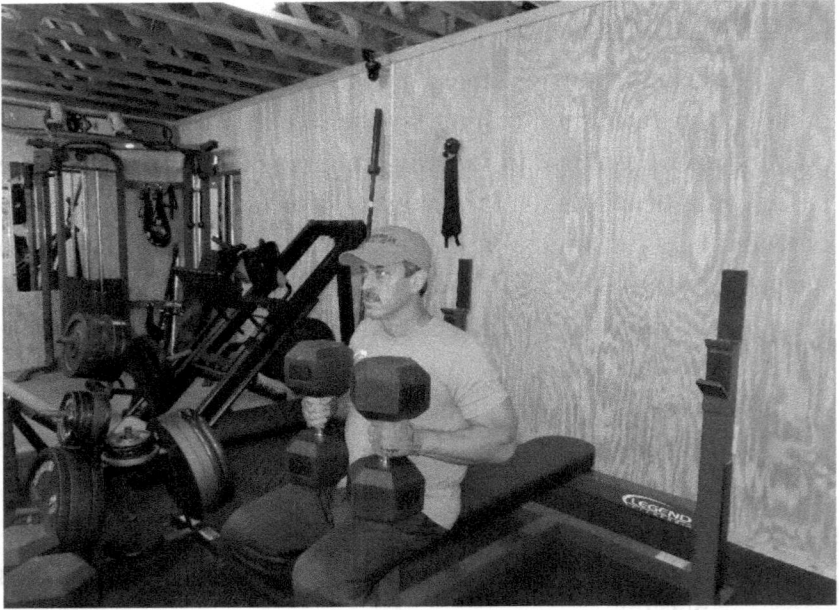

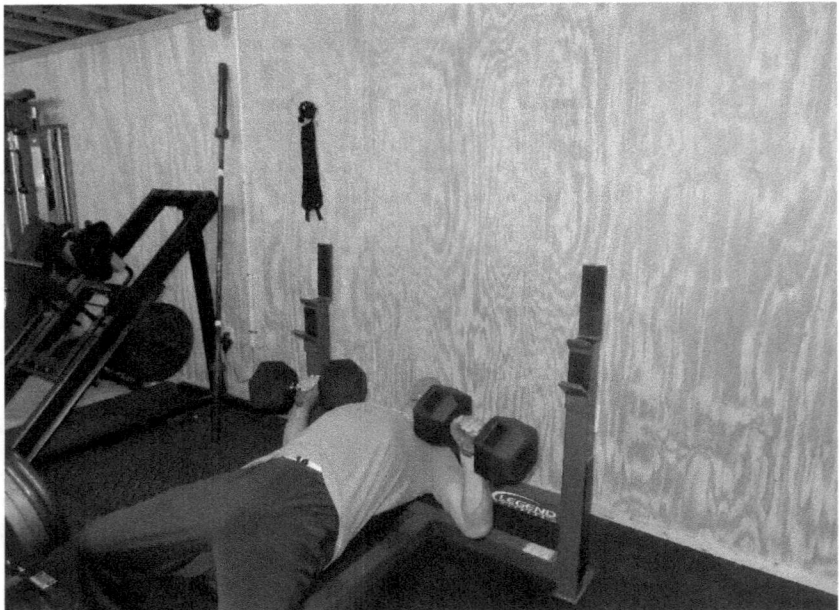

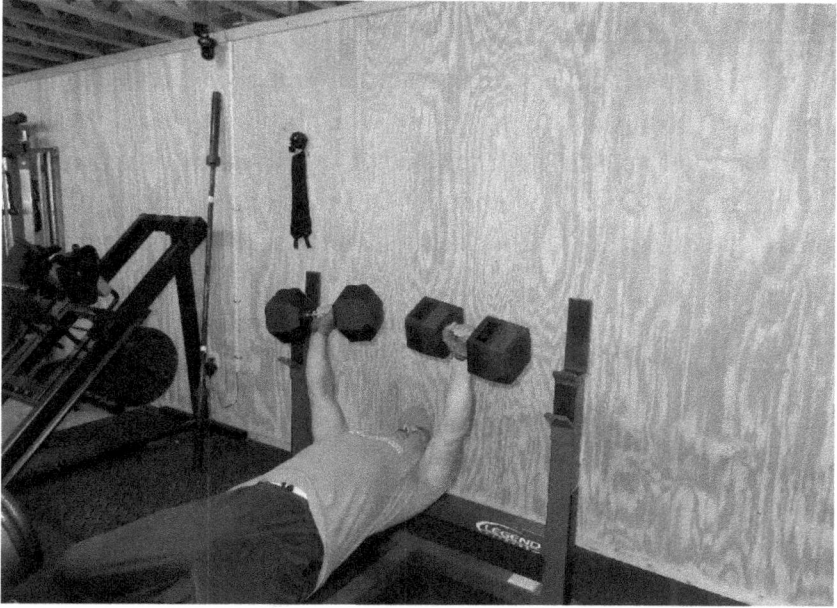

Dumbbell center press

Using a lighter weight than the dumbbell press, begin in the same position and manner. When you lie back, though, position your palms and the weights facing each other, and squeeze them firmly together. Then lift from the center of your torso, and bring the weights back down to the center of your torso.

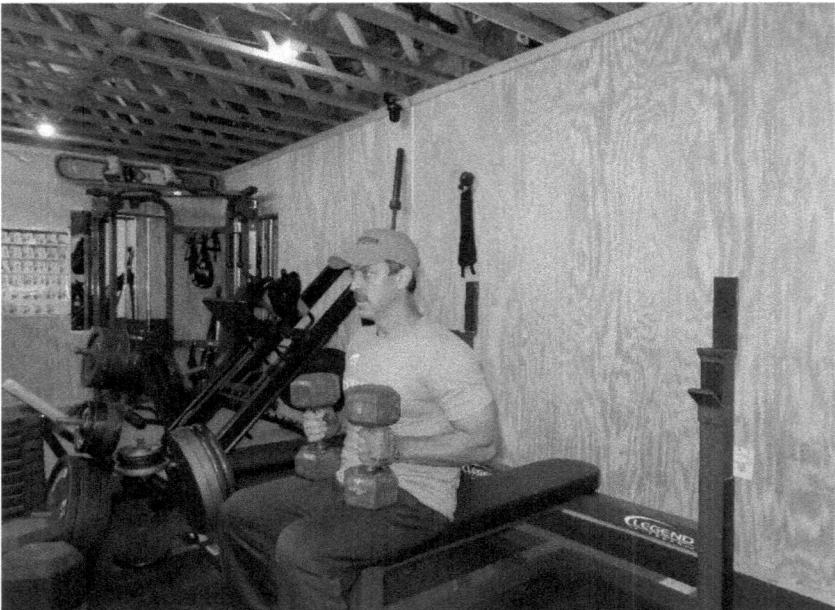

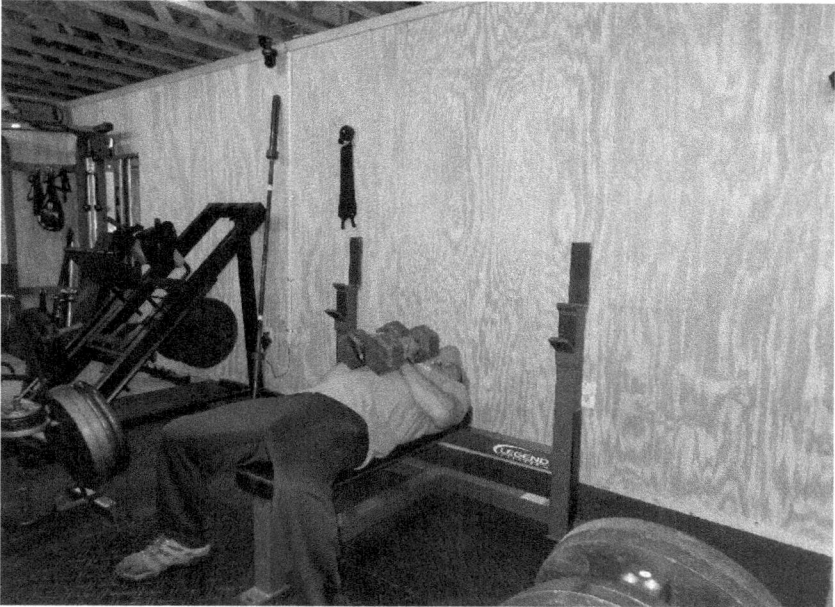

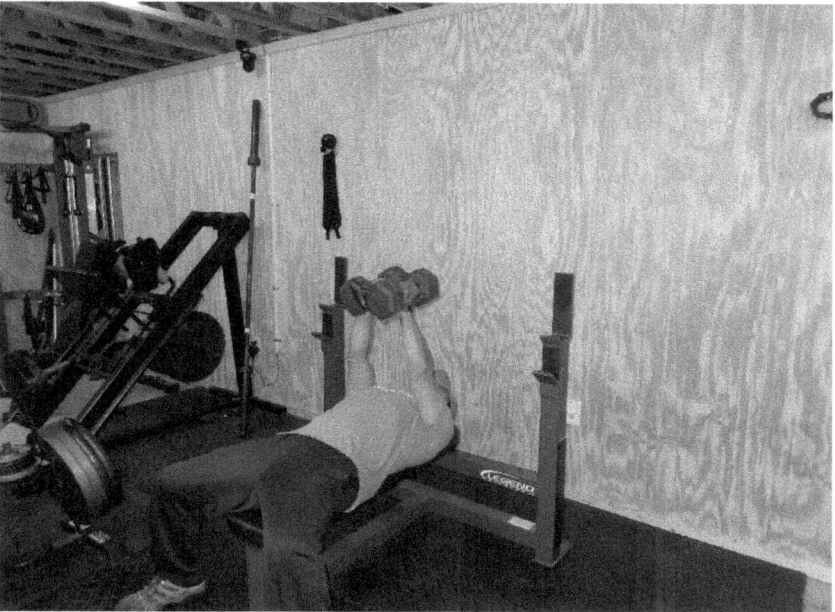

Cable flies

With the cable handles roughly chest high, bring them forward and to the center. Then in a controlled motion, keeping good tension, let the weights return to the starting point. Do not rush the return motion; if you will go a bit slower, your muscles will benefit from both the push and the return motions.

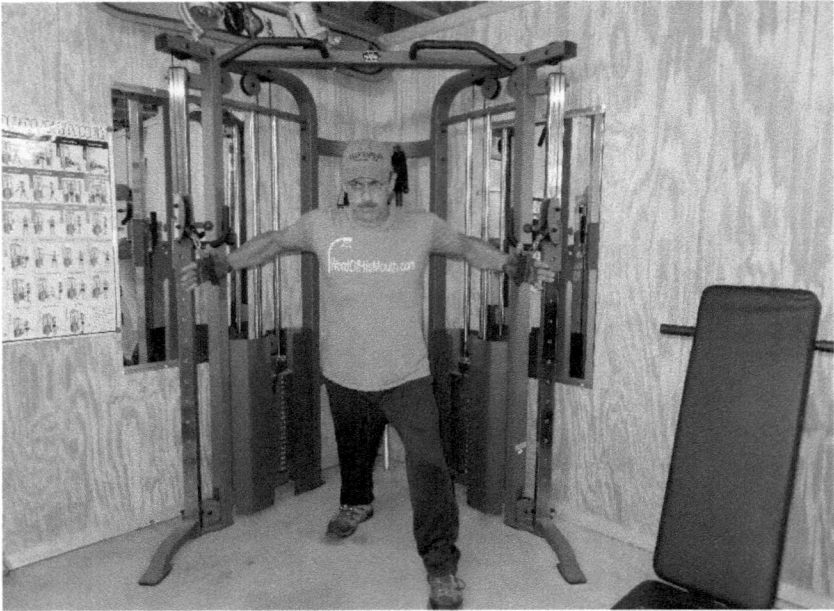

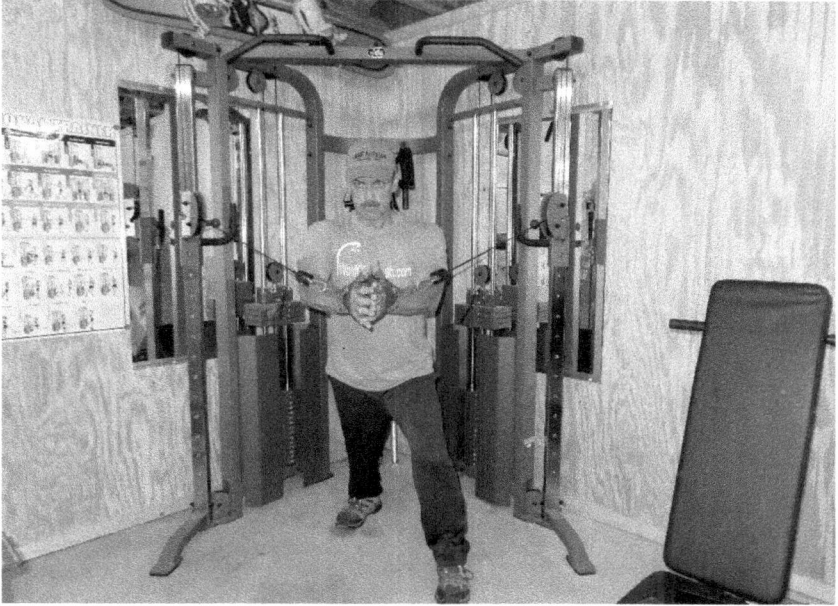

Pushups

Keep your back and body straight for the entire motion, and your hands roughly the same distance apart as when you bench press. You can also do the same motion with your hands just chest width apart, which, like the close-grip bench press, really hits your triceps.

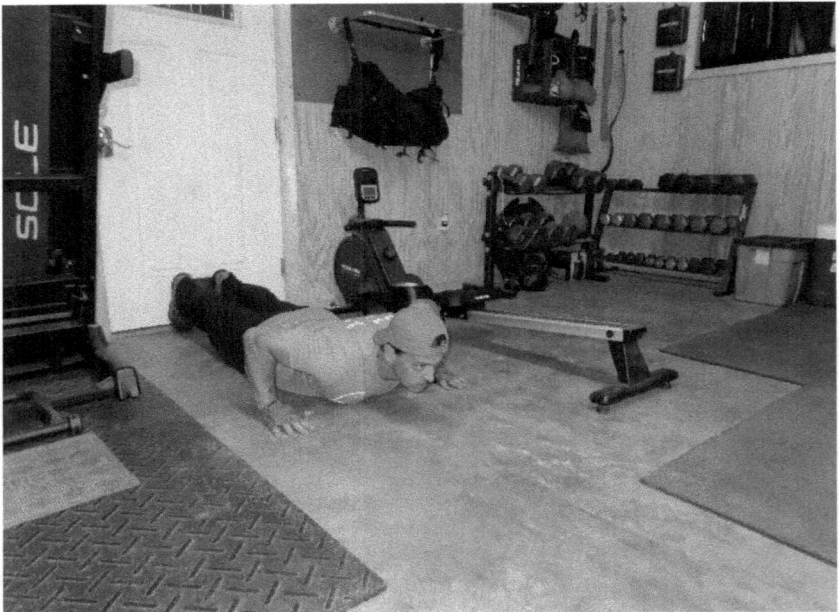

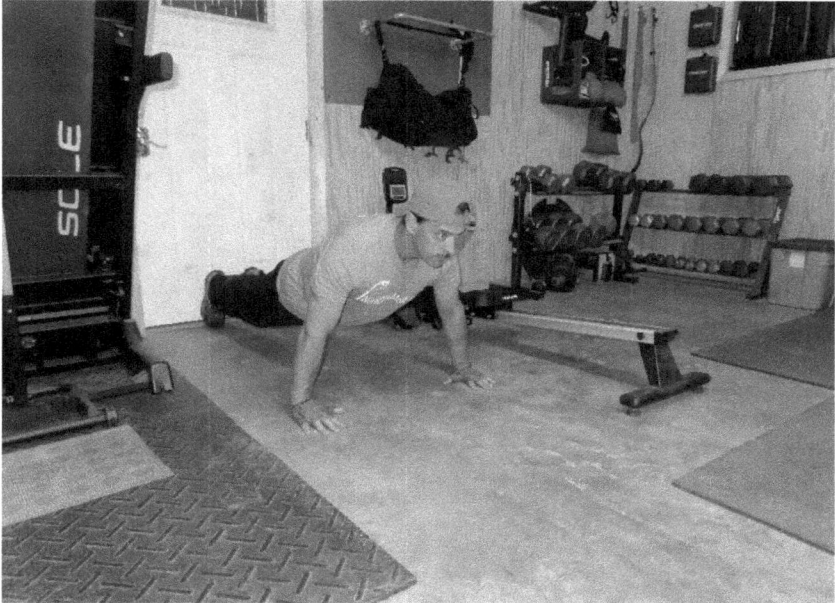

Narrow Grip Push Up

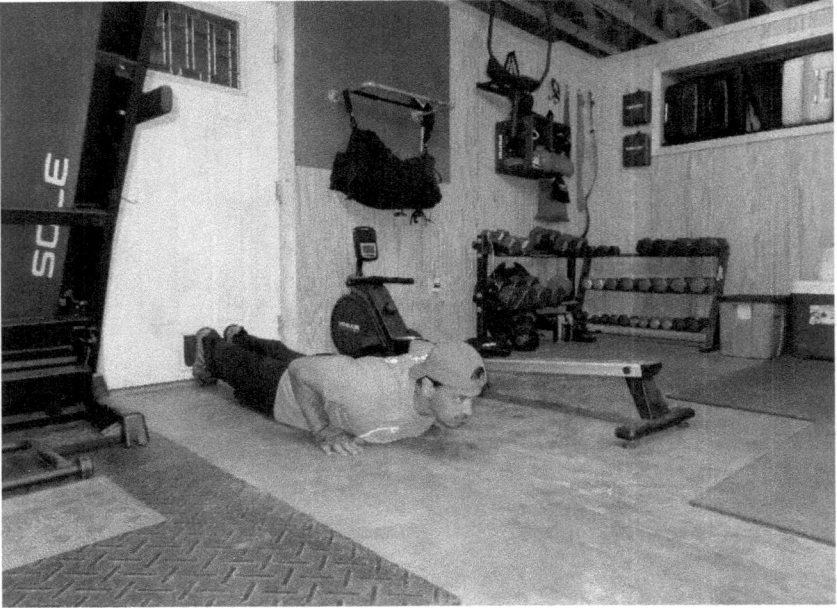

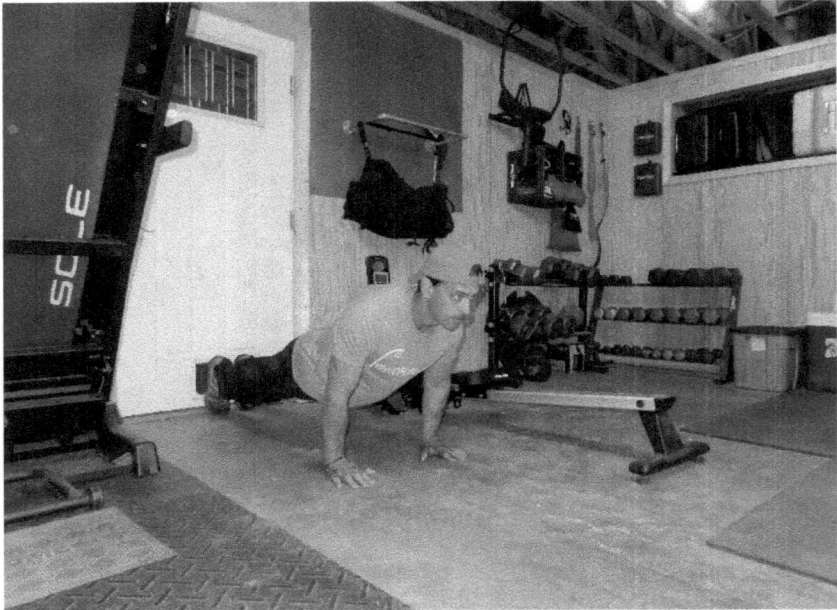

Clapping pushups   *Just for fun

Keep your back and body straight for the entire motion, and your hands roughly the same distance apart as when you bench press. Explode upward, clap, and return to the starting position.

Biceps

Close-Grip Chin-Ups

Grip the bar or handles with a supinated (palms facing you) grip. As much as possible, keep your body from swaying while you pull yourself upward and lower yourself downward.

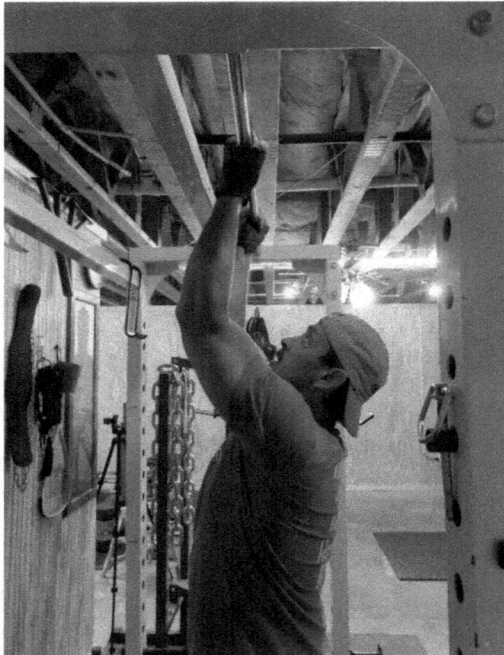

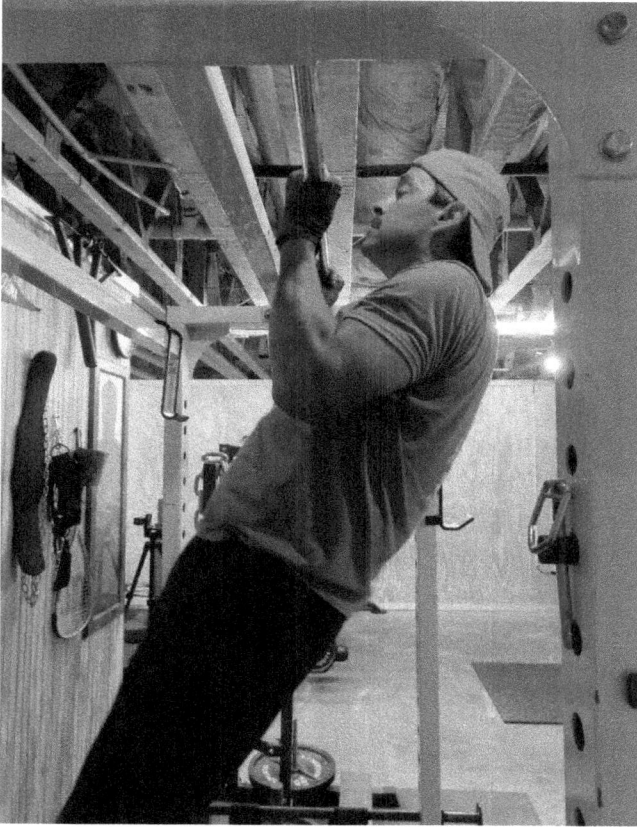

Hammer curl chin-ups

Grip the bar or handles with a hammer grip. As much as possible, keep your body from swaying while you pull yourself upward and lower yourself downward.

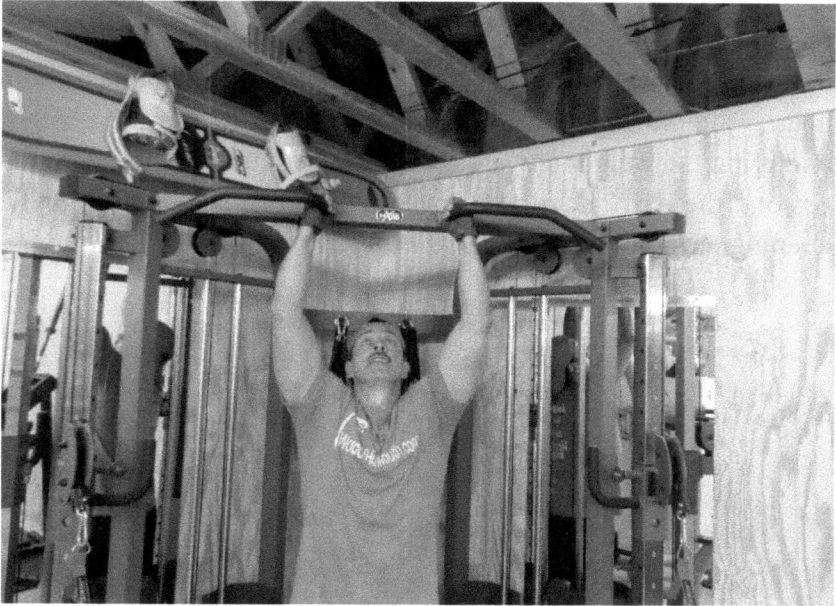

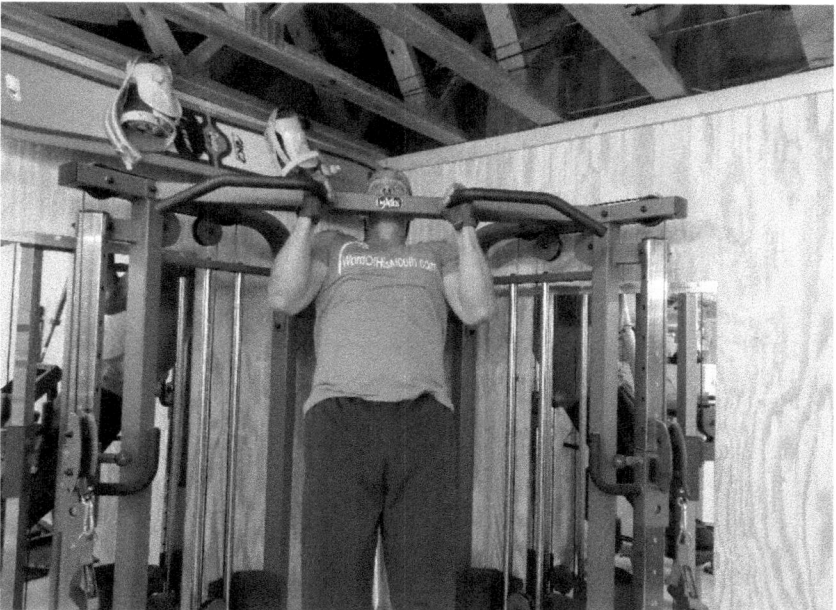

Barbell curls

Grip the bar with your hands roughly shoulder-width apart. Without swaying to gain momentum, lift from the biceps and bring the weight upward, pausing and squeezing for a second or so at the top. Then lower the weight down somewhat slowly, keeping tension on the biceps the entire time.

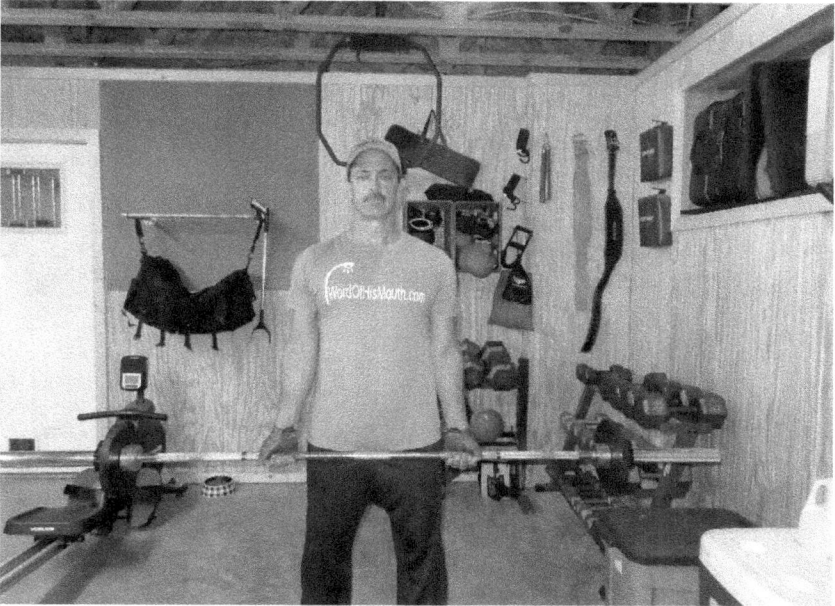

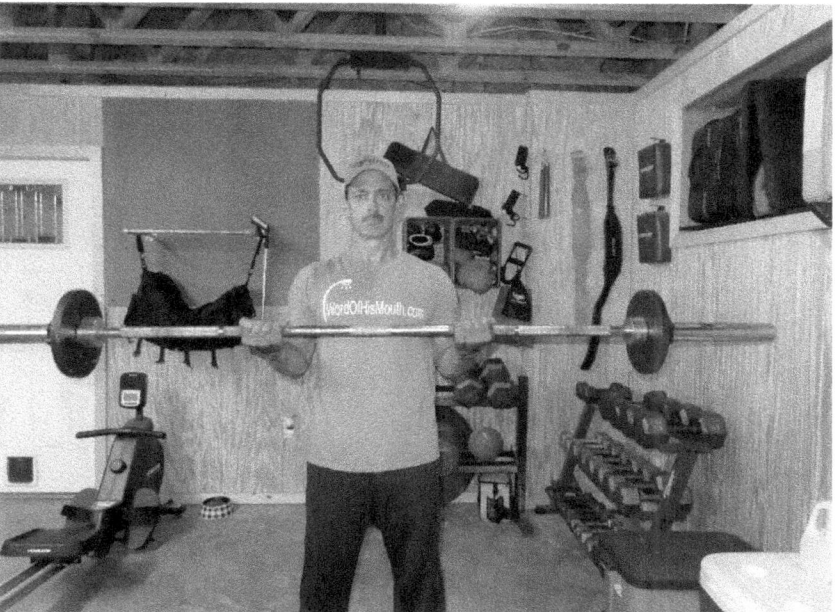

Reverse cable bicep curls

Set the cable and bar at the lowest possible setting. Grip the bar with a pronated (palms facing away from you) grip. Without swaying to gain momentum, lift from the biceps and bring the weight upward, pausing and squeezing for a second or so at the top. Then lower the weight down somewhat slowly, keeping tension on the biceps the entire time.

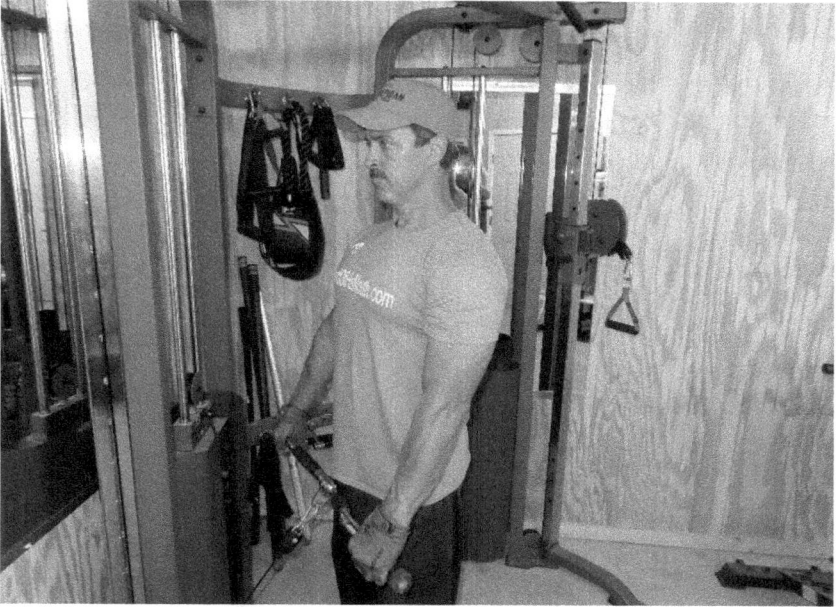

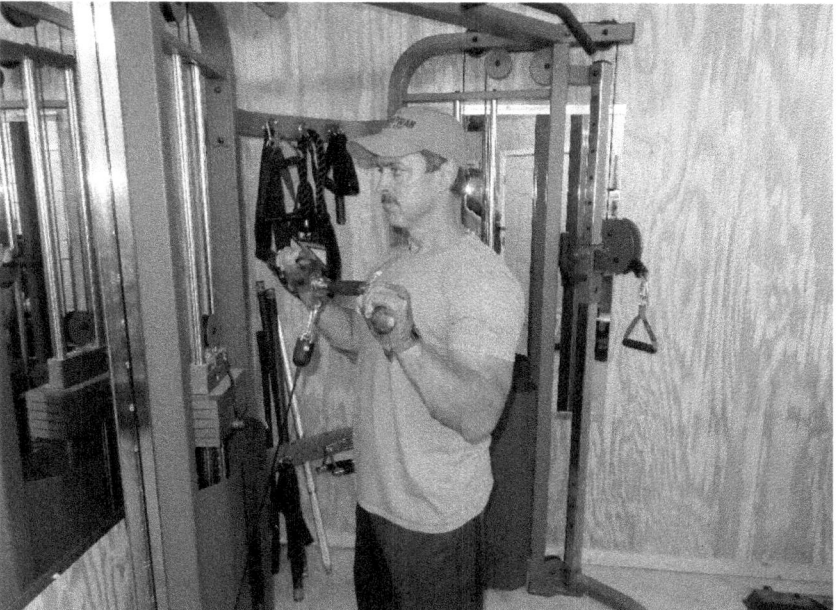

Wrist curls

      While seated on the bench, hold the barbell as wide apart as your knees are spread, resting your wrist on your knees, with your hands suspended in the air beyond your knees. Without engaging the shoulders, use your wrists and forearms to curl the bar as far as your wrists will allow, then come back down slowly.

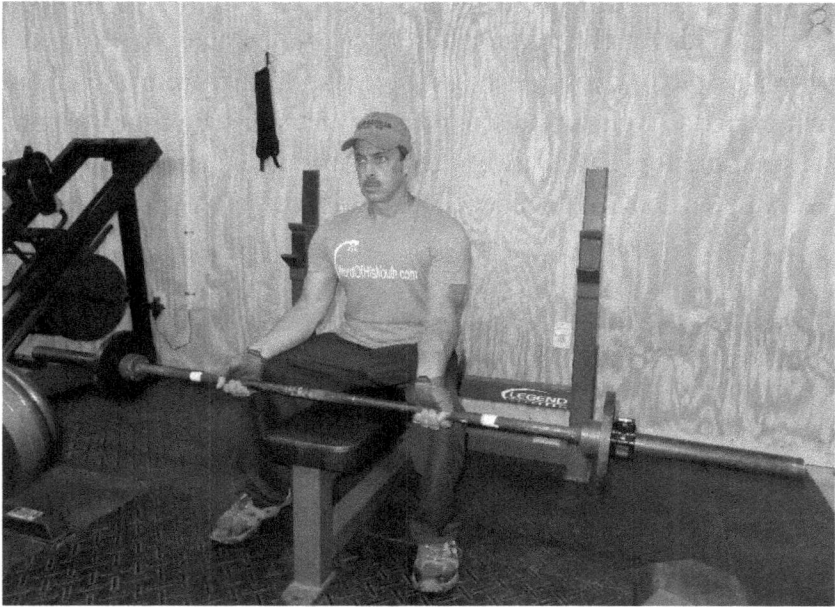

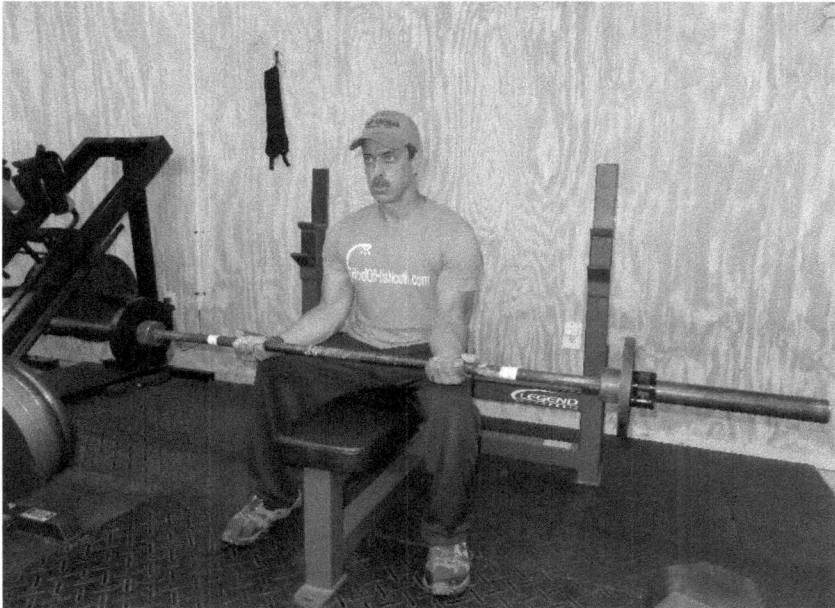

Dumbbell hammer curls

With your hands and dumbbell(s) in hammer position, and without swaying your body for momentum, lift from the biceps and bring the weight upward, pausing and squeezing for a second or so at the top. Then lower the weight down somewhat slowly, keeping tension on the biceps the entire time.

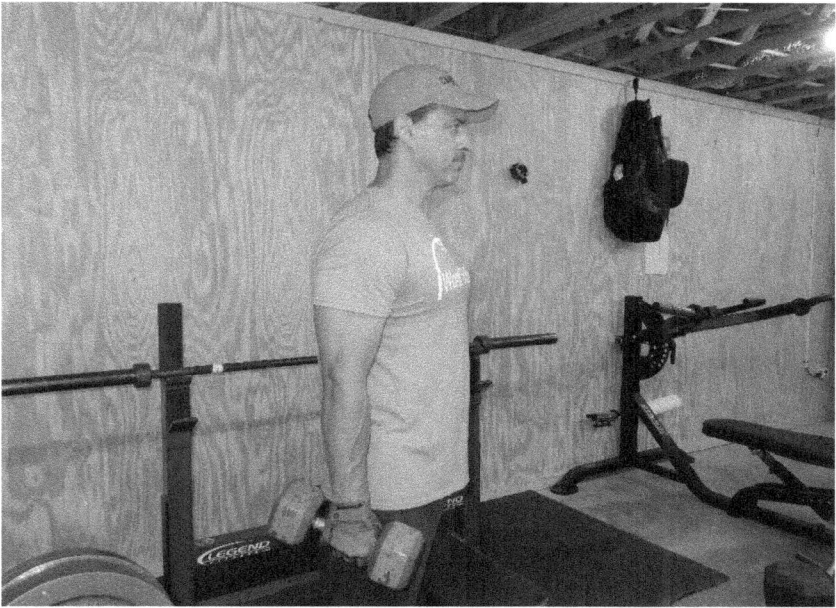

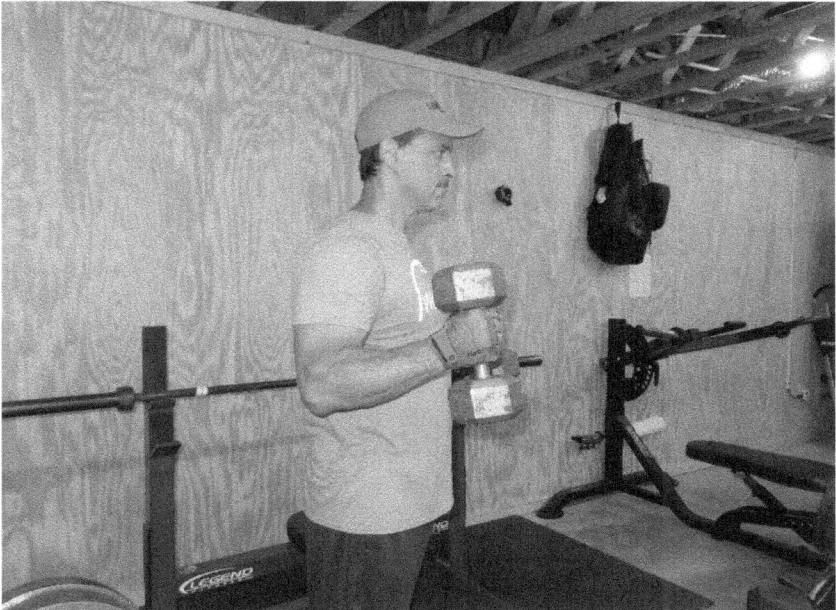

Easy Bar Curl

With your hands in a comfortable spot on the bar, and without swaying your body for momentum, lift from the biceps and bring the weight upward, pausing and squeezing for a second or so at the top. Then lower the weight down somewhat slowly, keeping tension on the biceps the entire time.

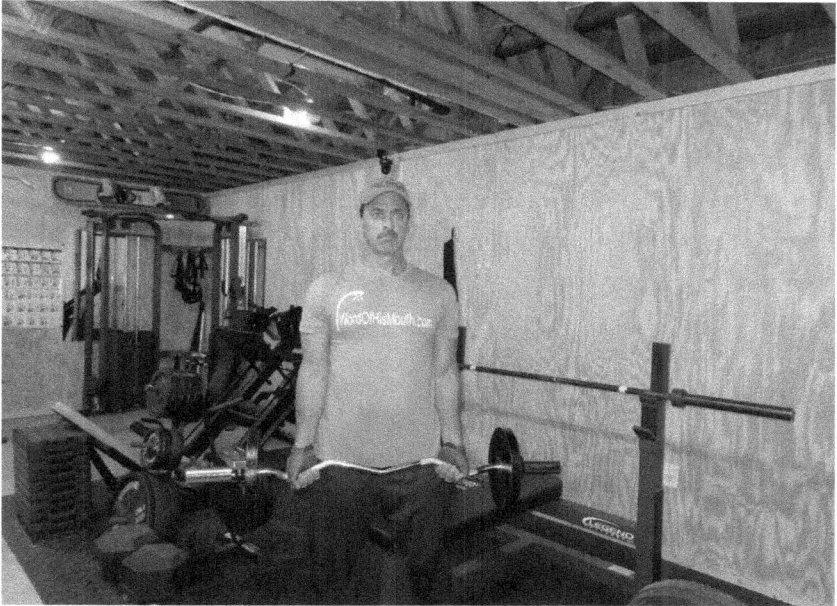

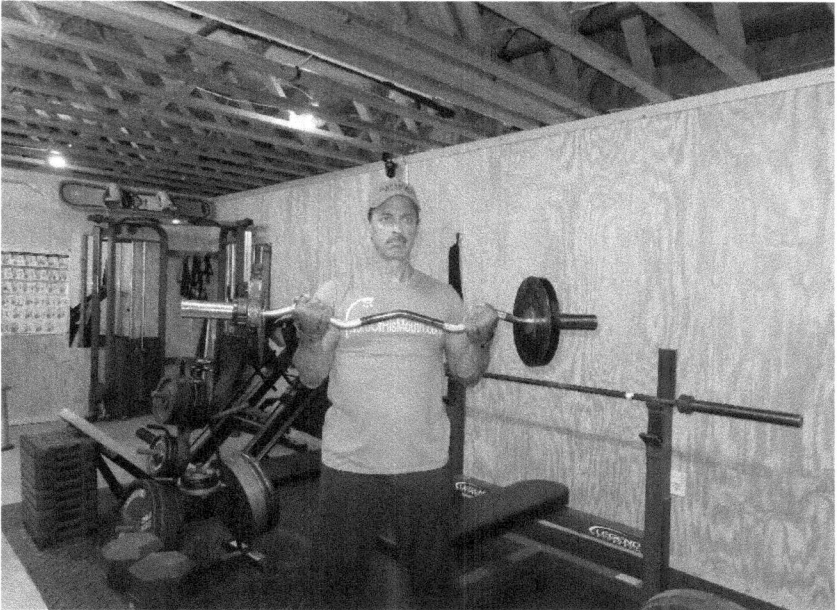

Seated chin-up. *Just for fun

Sitting cross-legged or with your legs straight out, use the power rack and a barbell. Grip the bar in a narrow grip with your palms facing you as you sit on the ground. Make sure the bar height requires you to stretch upward as high as you are able to grab it. Then lift yourself up to a full chin-up, and slowly lower yourself back down to the ground.

Triceps

<u>Dips</u>

With your hands on the supports on either side, and without swaying and rocking during the movement, lower your body to the lowest comfortable level, and then push back upward to full extension.

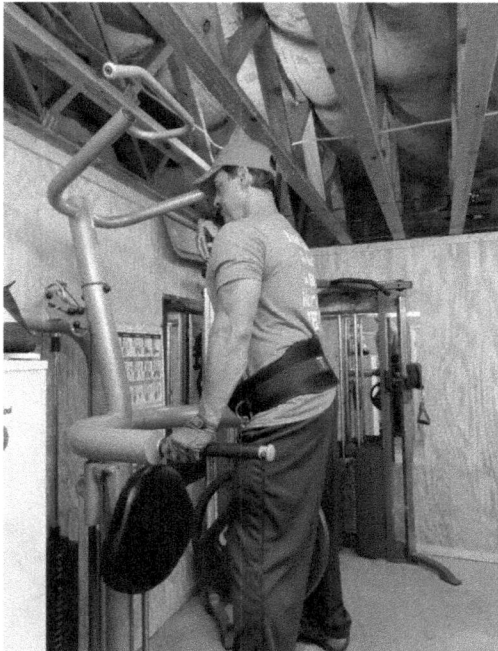

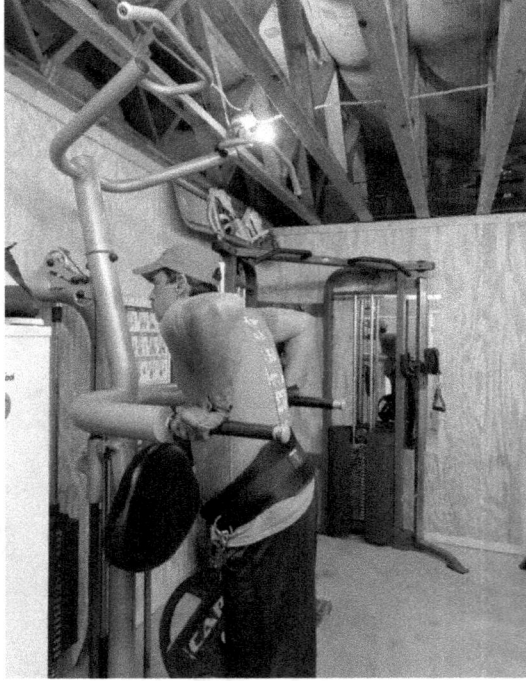

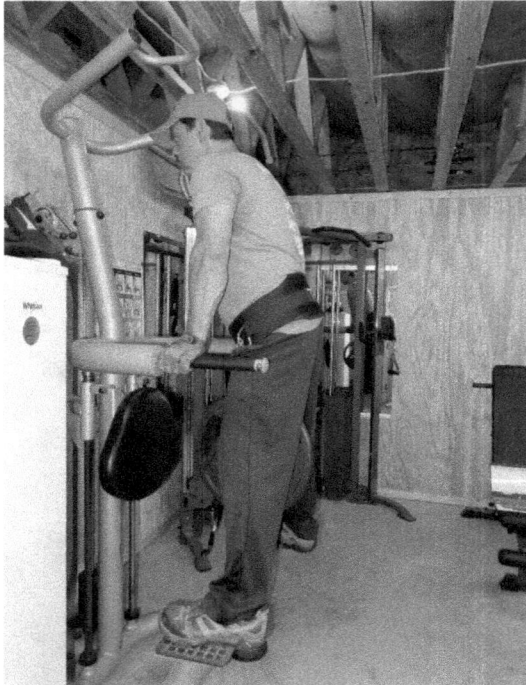

Close-grip bench press

With your elbows tucked in beside your chest, grip the bar. Have a spotter help with the liftoff. In a controlled manner, lower the bar to your chest, and then push back upward to full extension.

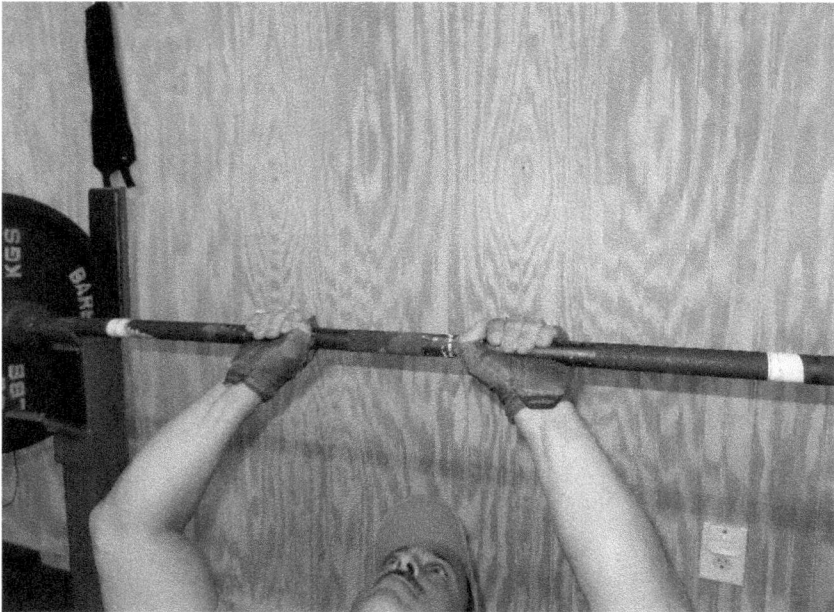

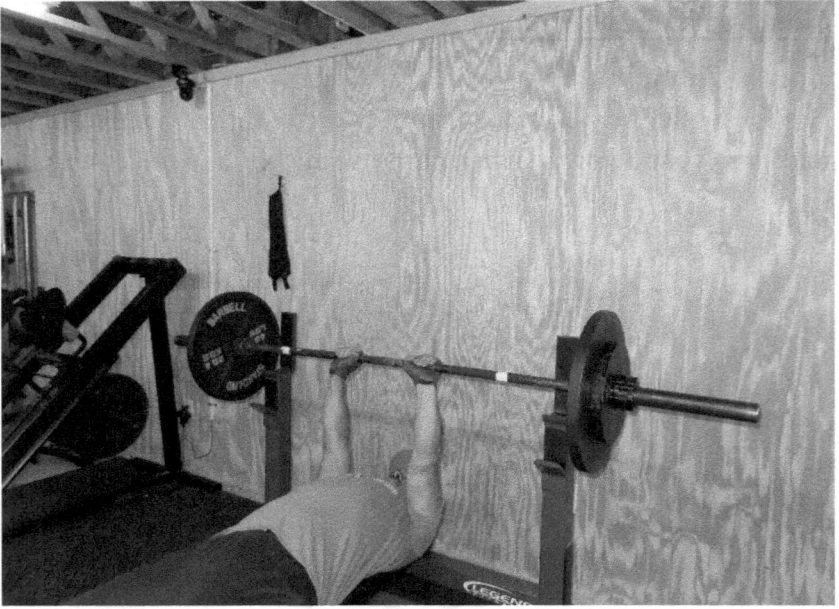

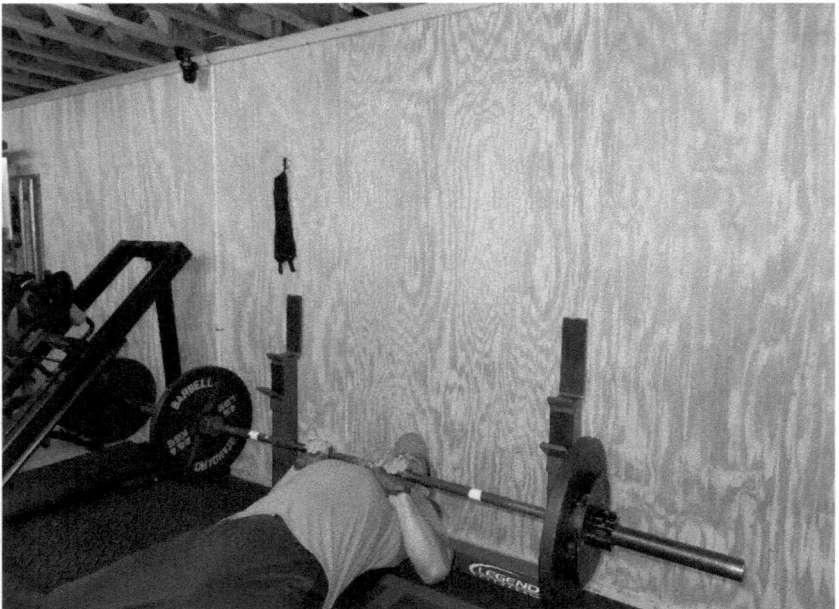

Rope pulls

With your upper body angled slightly forward, grip either side of the rope, pull down, and flare at the bottom. Return the weight in a slow, controlled manner. Continue to do this to failure, and then do as many more reps as possible with your hands pressed together.

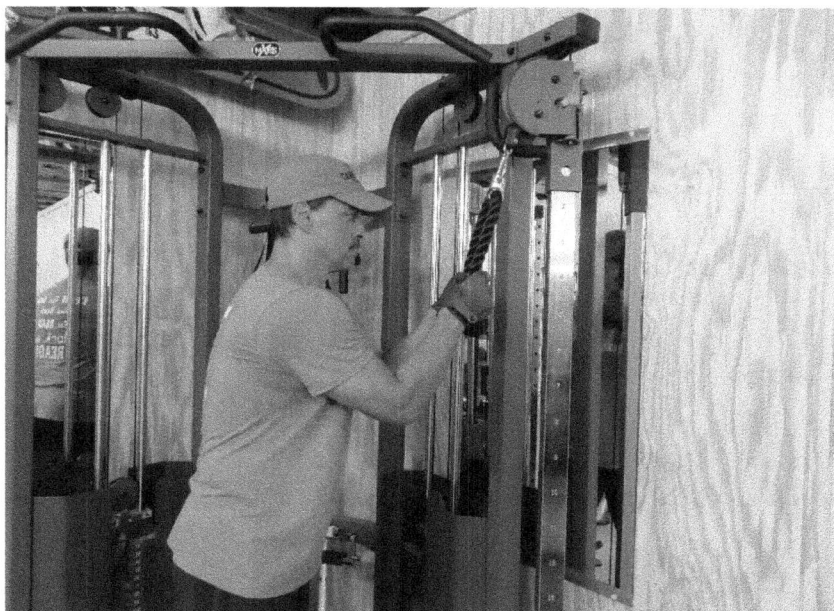

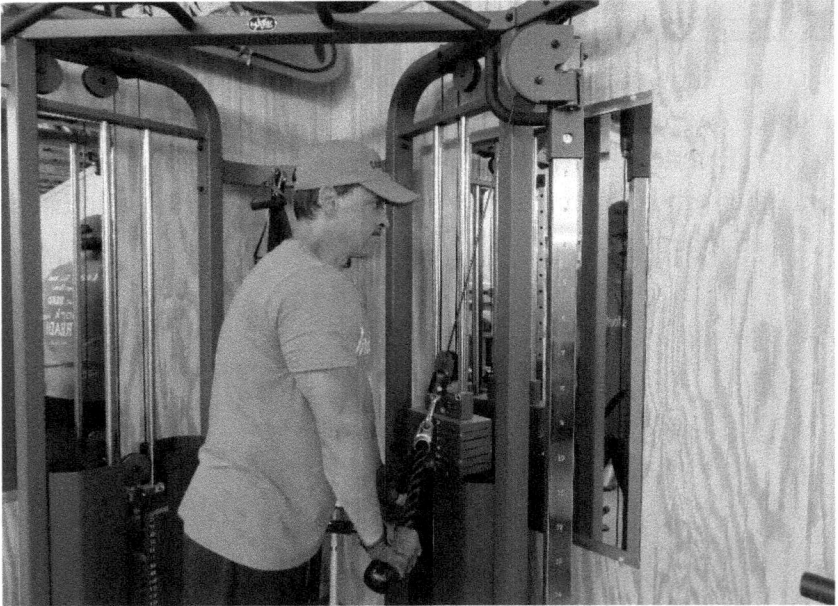

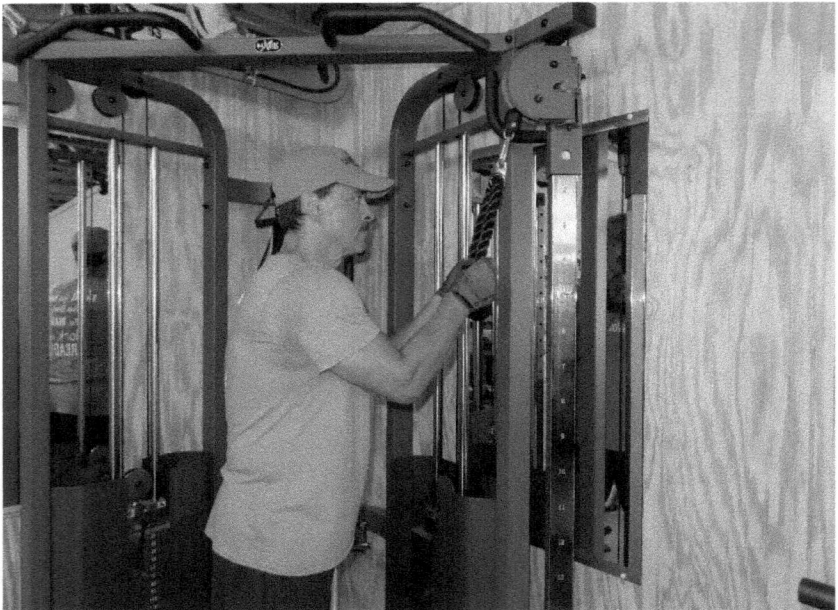

Bar push down

With your upper body angled slightly forward and your thumbs on top of the bar, push the bar down as if trying to roll it through your body. Return the weight in a slow, controlled manner.

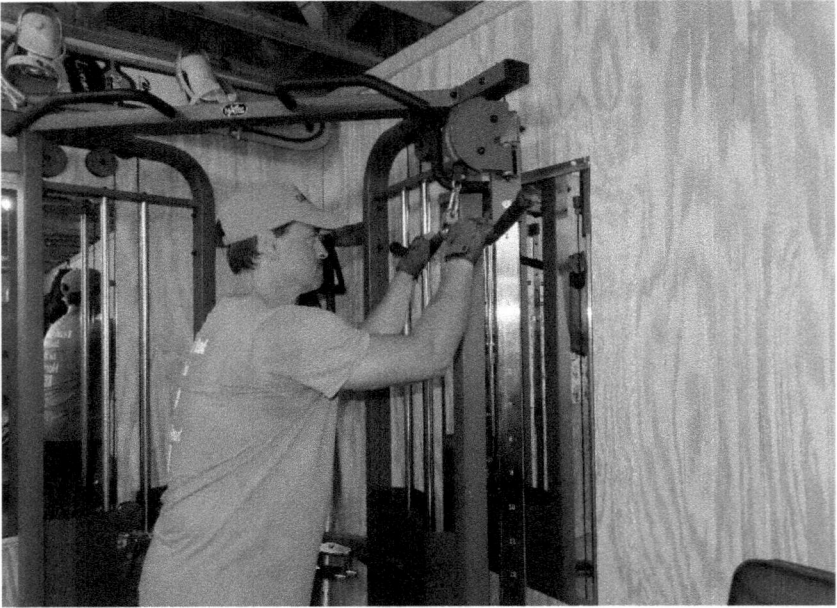

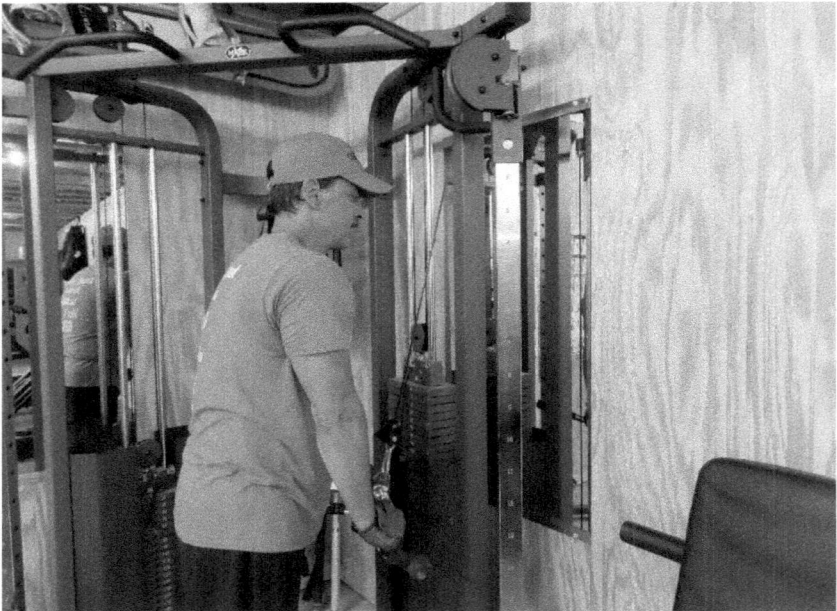

Well pumps

With the cable set roughly chest high, position the bar directly under your chest, and push down from the top. Depending on the machine, you can either have the cable wheel beneath your chin or have the cable itself come down beside your face. Return the weight in a slow, controlled manner.

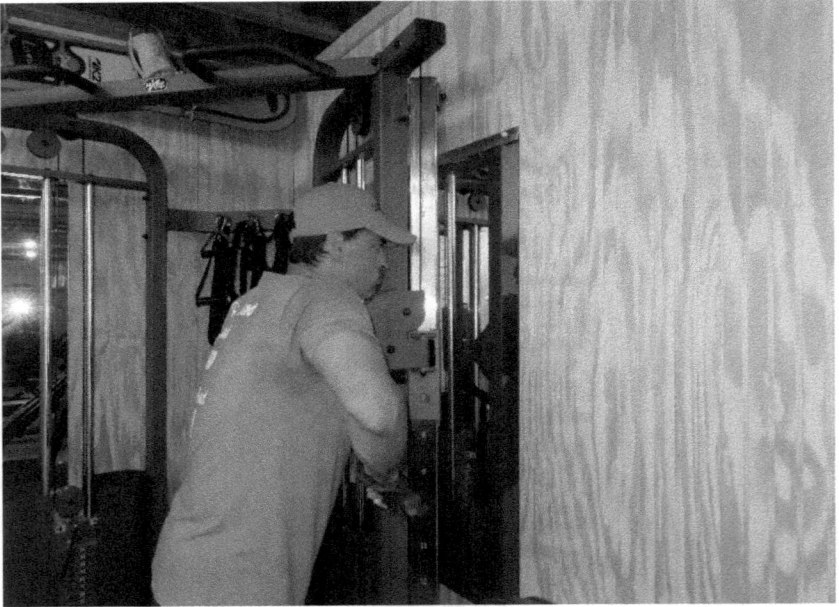

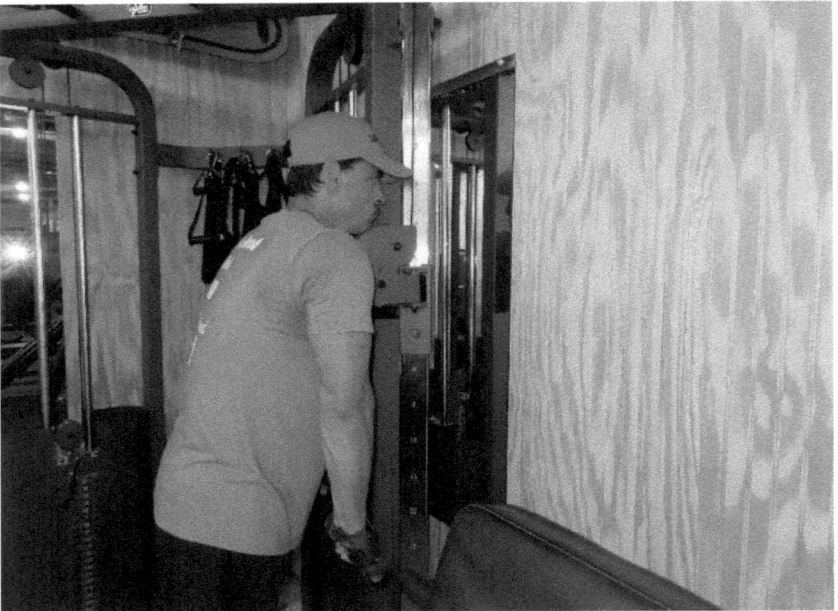

Reverse triceps curls

With the cable wheel at the highest position, grip the bar in an underhanded position. Then flex it down and back toward your body, squeezing the triceps at the bottom of the motion for a second. Return the weight in a slow, controlled manner.

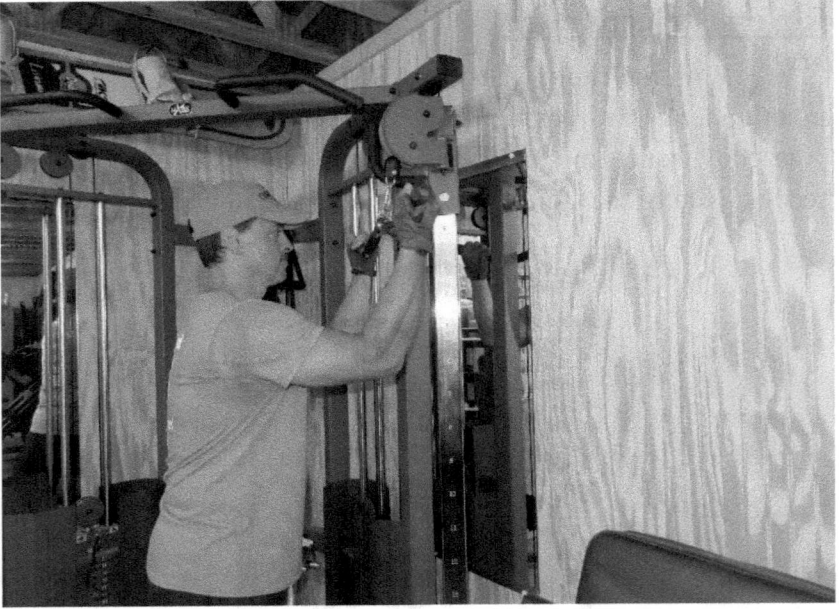

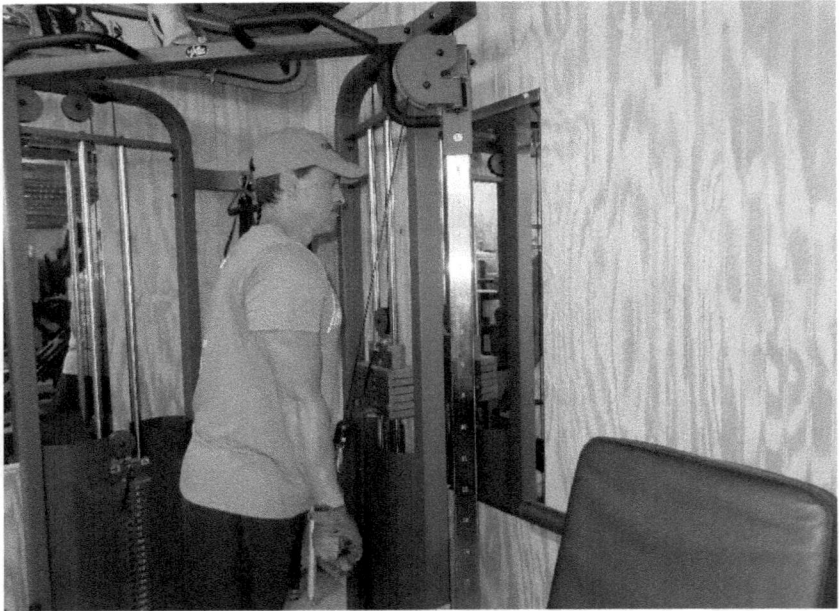

Overhead rope pulls

With the rope and pulley in a high position, grip the rope from behind your head, and lean forward. Then extend your arms outward, and then return the weight in a slow, controlled manner.

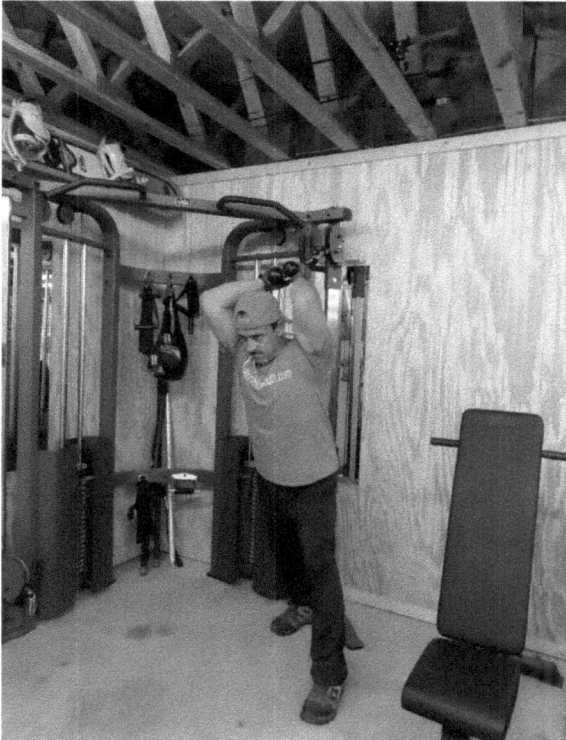

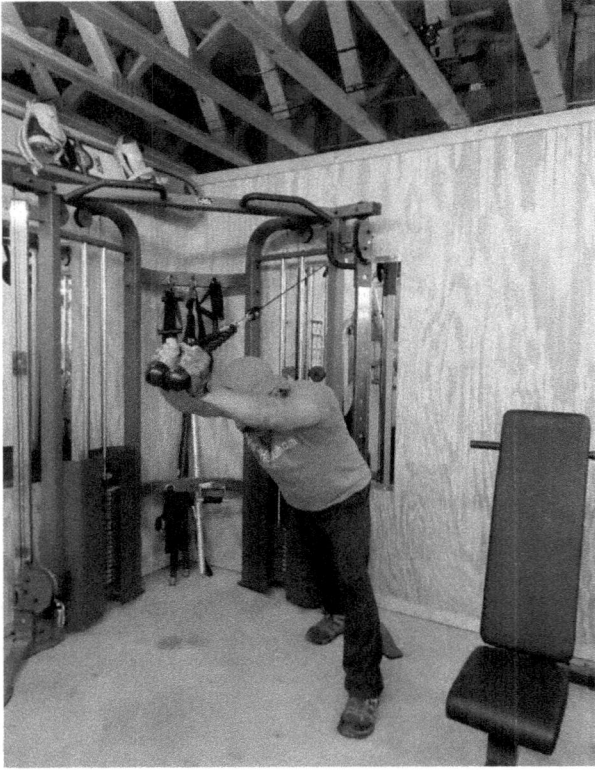

One-arm pushups   *Just for fun

With one arm and hand under the center of your chest, and your body cocked at a slight angle, put your other arm behind your back, and push yourself up, then slowly lower yourself back down to the ground.

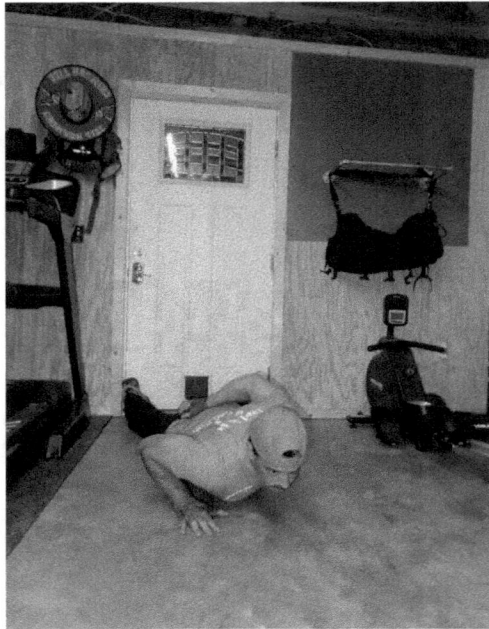

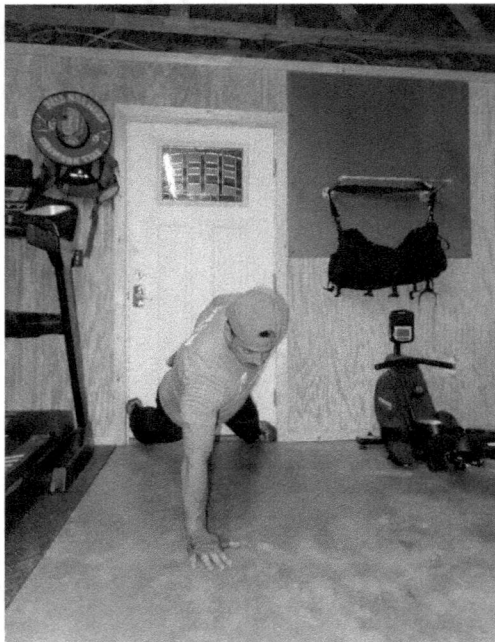

Back

<u>Wide grip pull-ups</u>

With your palms facing away from you, and with as wide a grip as possible, pull yourself upward, squeezing your shoulder blades toward each other at the top. Lower yourself back to the starting position in a slow, controlled manner.

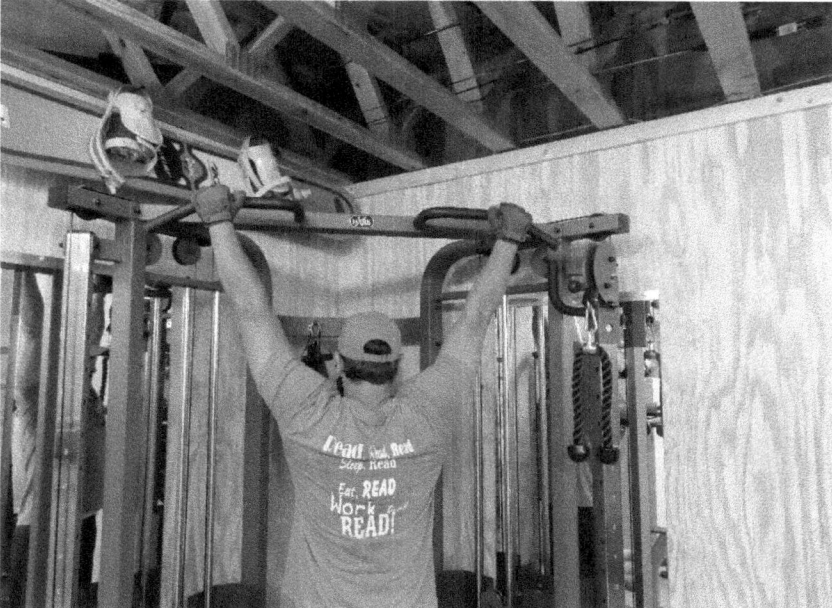

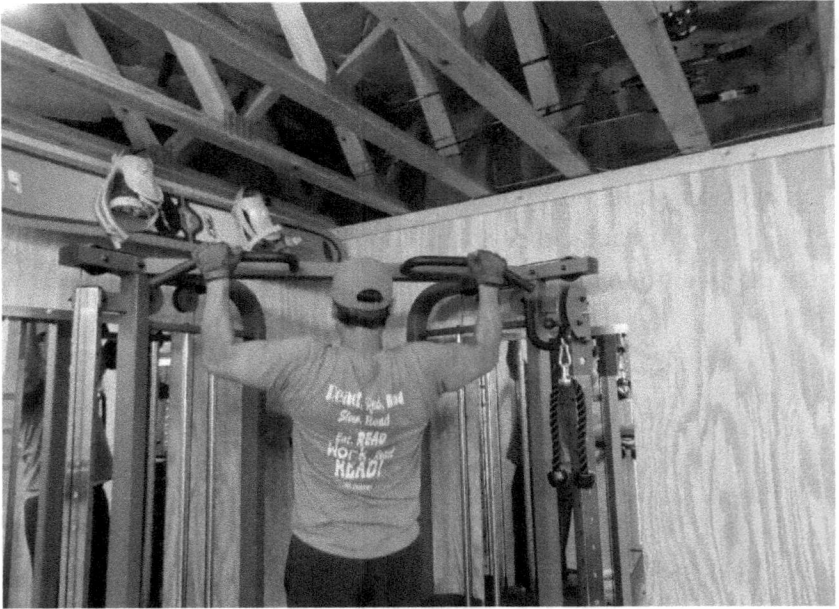

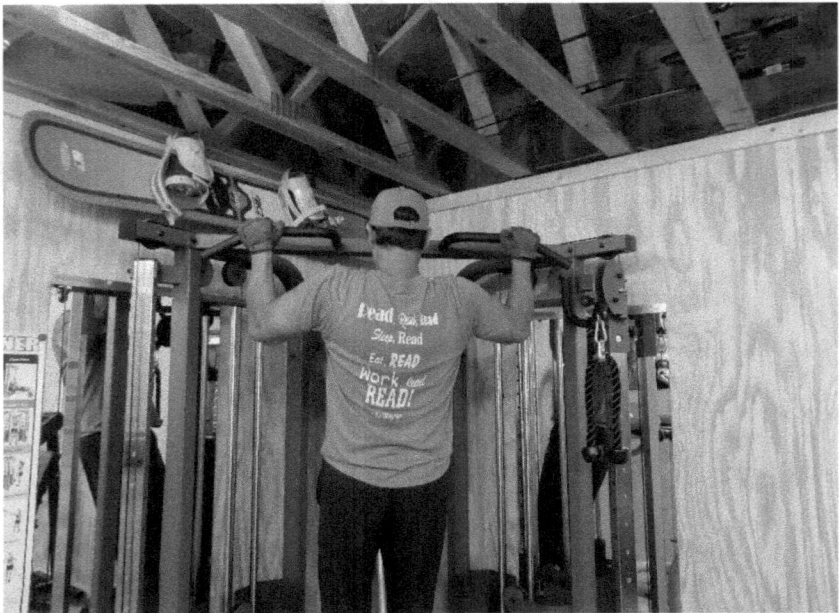

Stiff-legged dead lifts

Keeping your legs very straight, bend your body over from the waist, raise your body and the weight up until you are standing straight up, then, still keeping your legs straight, lower the weight in a slow, controlled manner.

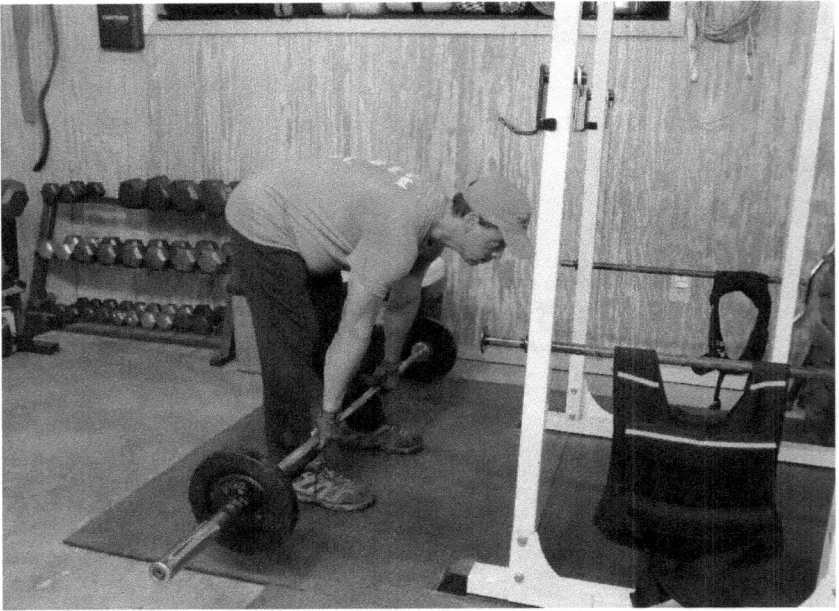

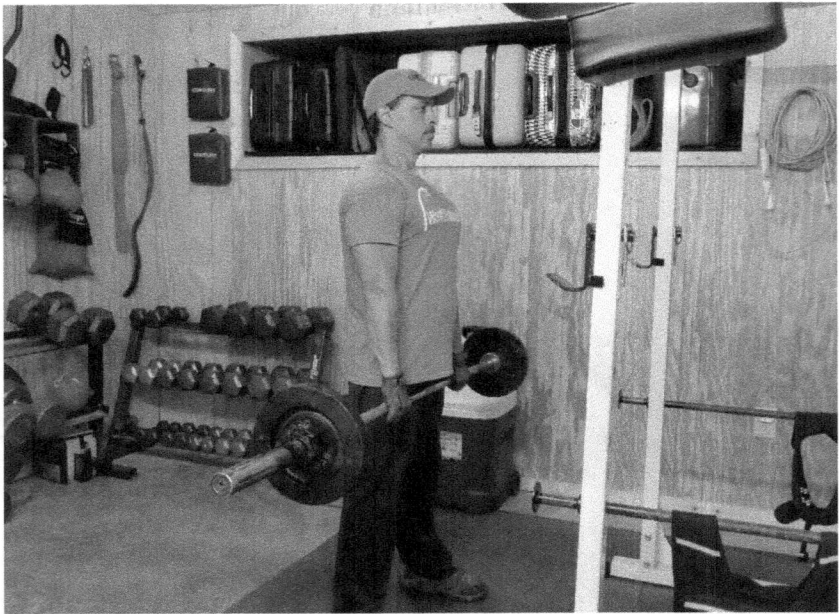

Lat pull-downs

With the bar and cable in the highest position, sit facing the cable and hold the bar with your palms facing away from you. Grip the bar in a wide position. Without jerking, pull it down to your upper chest, squeeze, and return to the starting position in a slow, controlled manner.

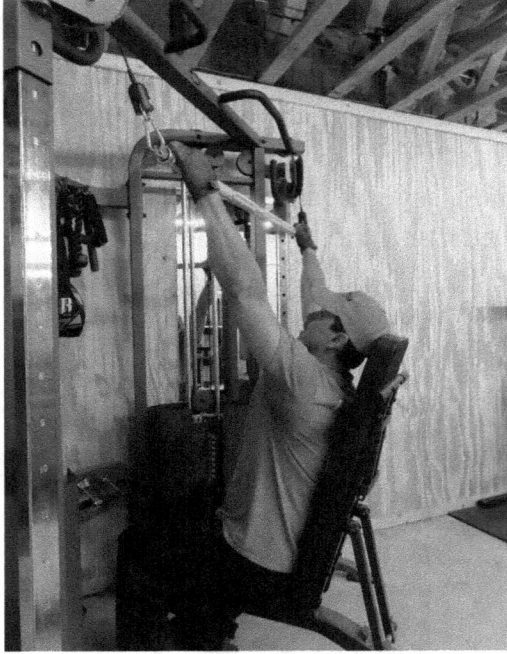

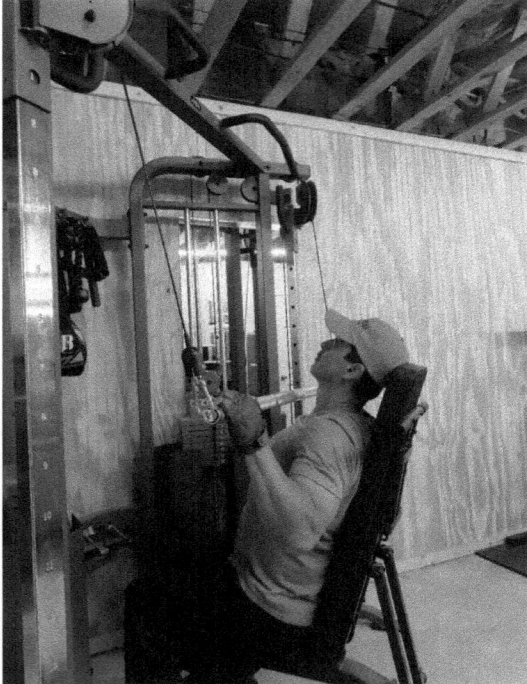

Narrow grip lat pull-downs

Position the cable to the highest position. Sit facing the machine. With your palms facing away from you, grip the bar in a narrow position. Without jerking, pull it down to your upper chest, squeeze, and return to the starting position in a slow, controlled manner.

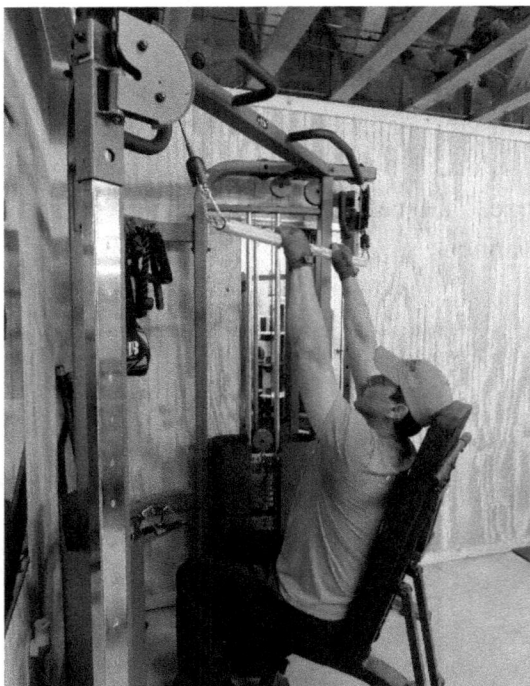

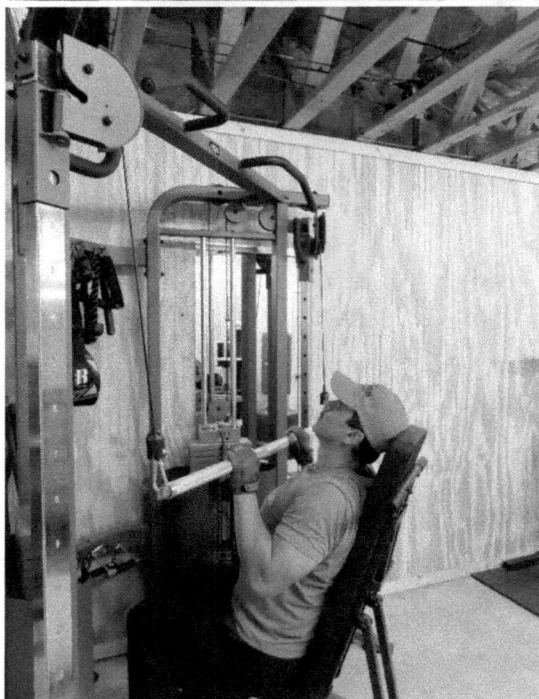

114

Stiff arm bar push down

With the bar in a high position, extend your arms straight outward, and put your hands and thumbs on top of the bar. Pivot your entire arms downward as if trying to roll them and the bar through and past your body. Then return the weight in a slow, controlled manner.

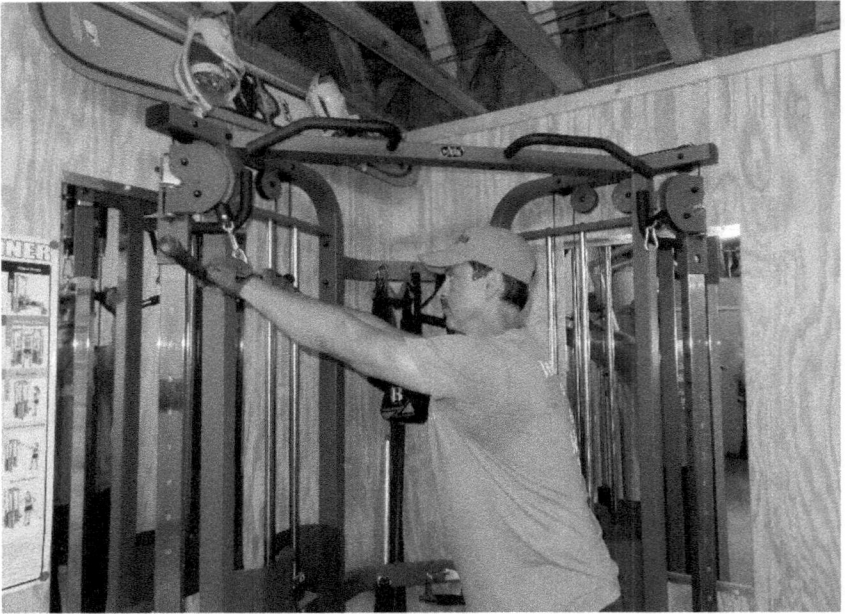

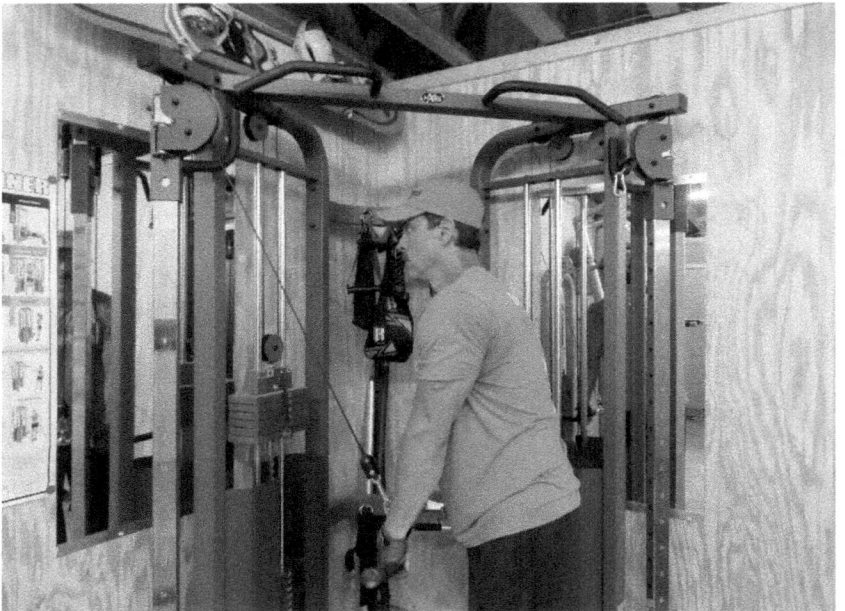

Low row

Set the cable to the lowest position and sit facing the machine. Lean forward and grab the handle, then pull yourself back into an upright position. *Maintaining a full upright position, let the weight slowly pull your arms out to full extension, and then pull your hands and the handle back to your body.

*Others prefer to lean their body over with each extension. I personally prefer it my way.

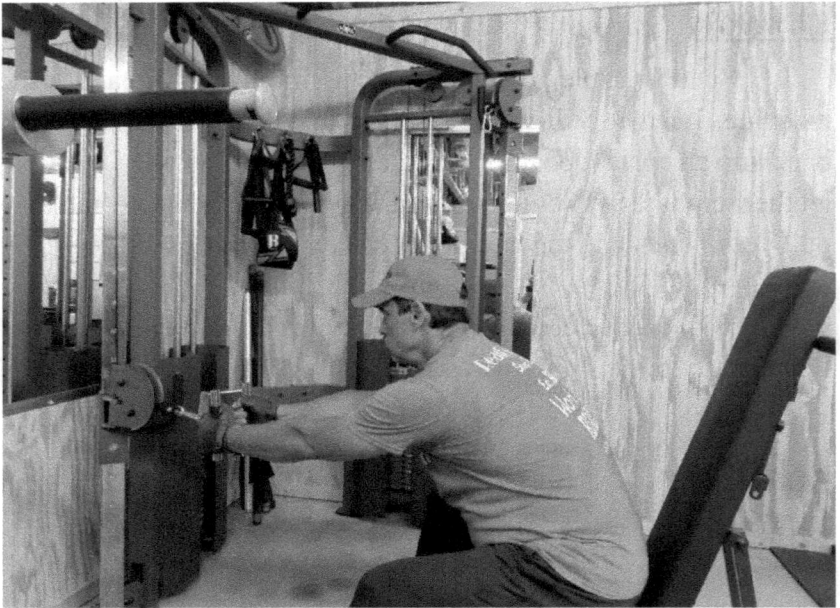

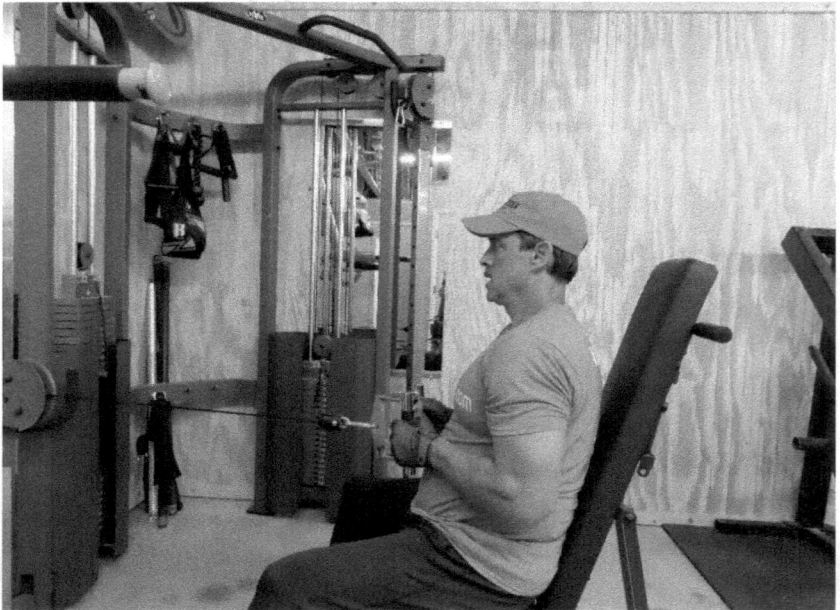

Dante row

With the rope in a low position, and either with or without a bench in front of you, bend your upper body forward ninety degrees or so. Grip the rope with your arms fully extended, and pull your hands back to your sides. Then return the rope and weight in a slow, controlled manner.

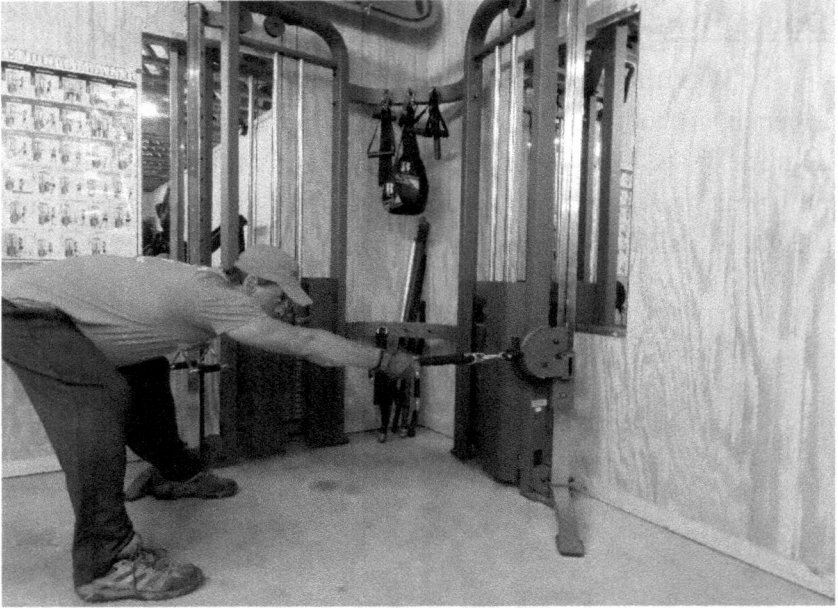

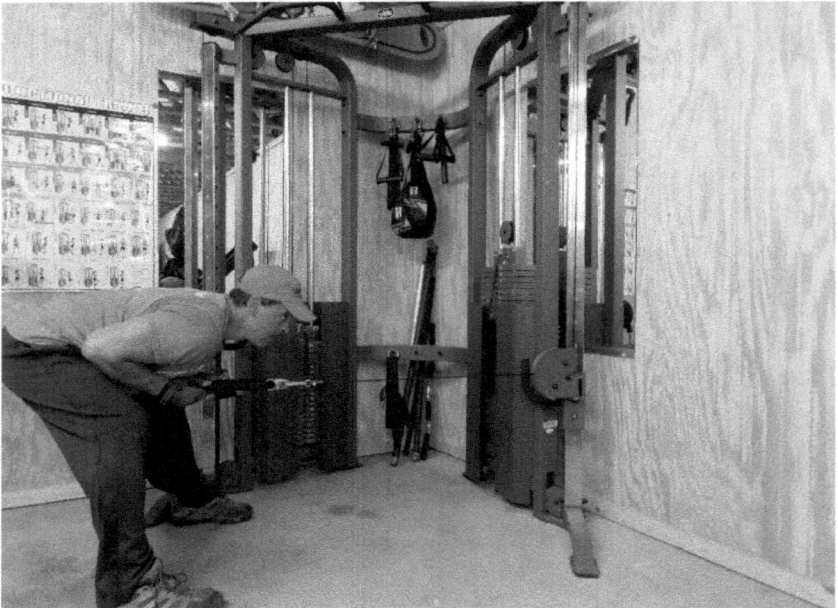

Bar twist

With the cable about ½ way up, turn the bar upright, one hand high on the bar, one hand low on the bar, twist your body away from the tension, and then let the tension slowly pull you back to the starting position.

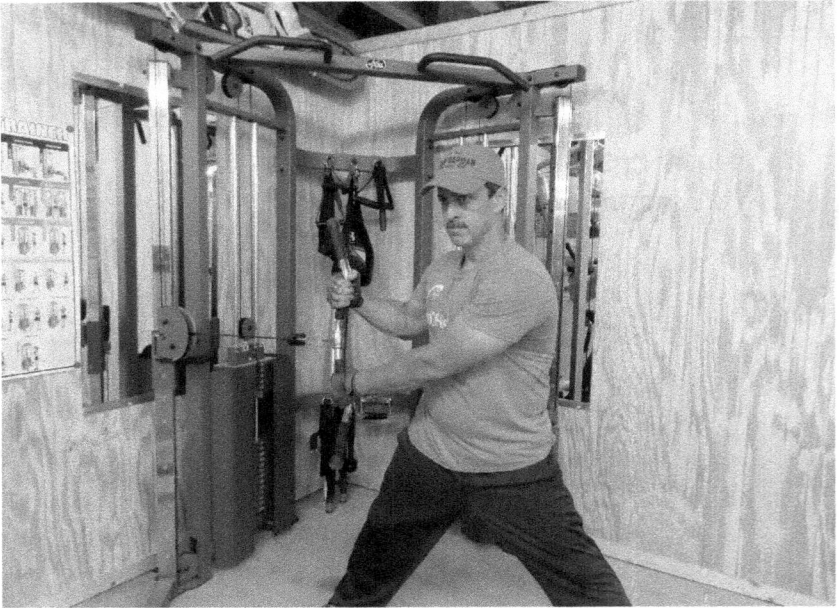

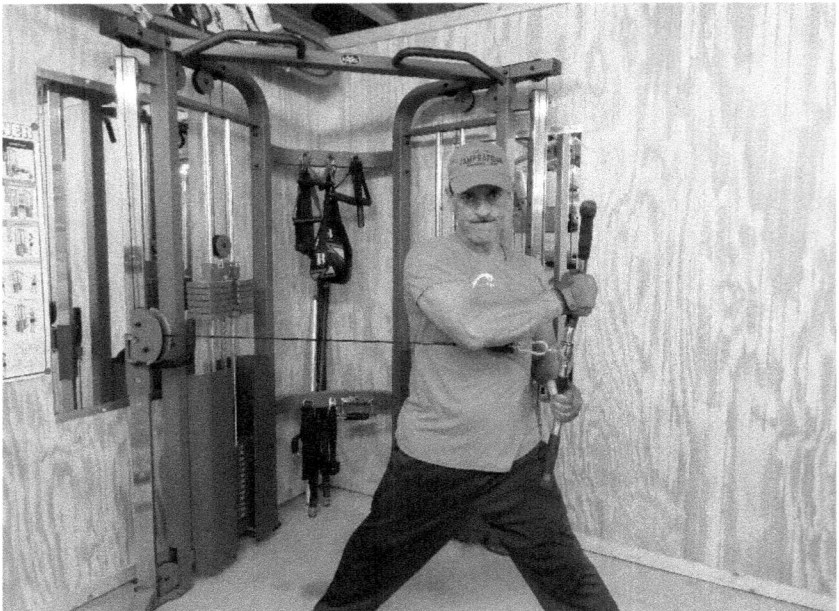

Pull up seated raises.   *Just for fun

Using the power rack and a barbell, sit either cross-legged or straight-legged with your hands in the pronated position (palms facing away from you). Pull yourself up, and in a slow, controlled manner, lower yourself down again.

Shoulders

Behind the head shoulder press

With your hands at a safe and comfortable width, put your traps under the bar, and stand upright to lift it off the rack. Take a step back, then push the weight upward. Lower it down, but only to about 90 degrees.

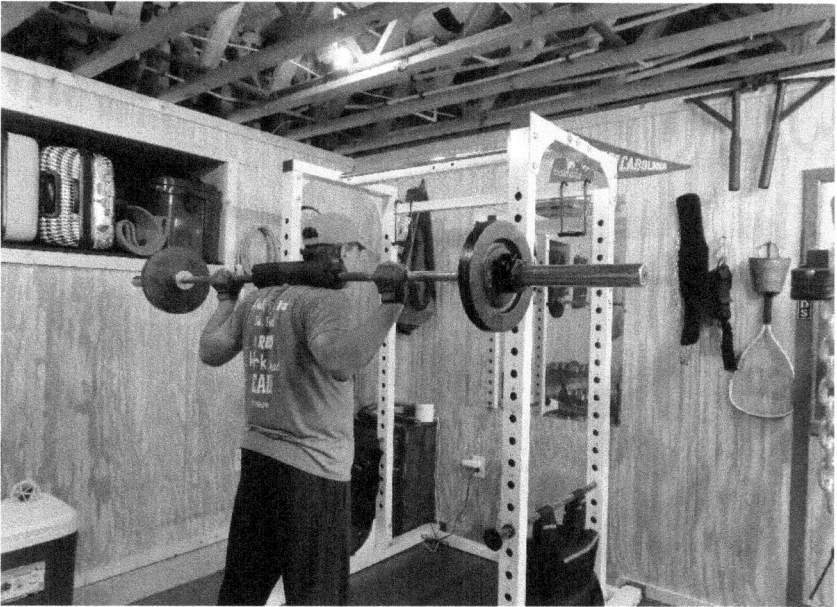

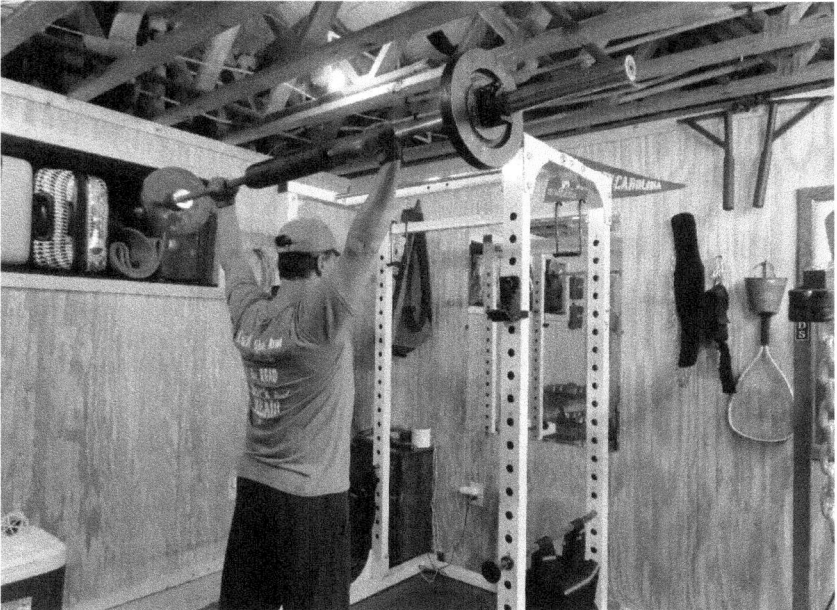

Machine shoulder press

With the handles at a safe and comfortable height, push the handles upward to nearly full extension, then lower the weight back down again in a slow, controlled manner.

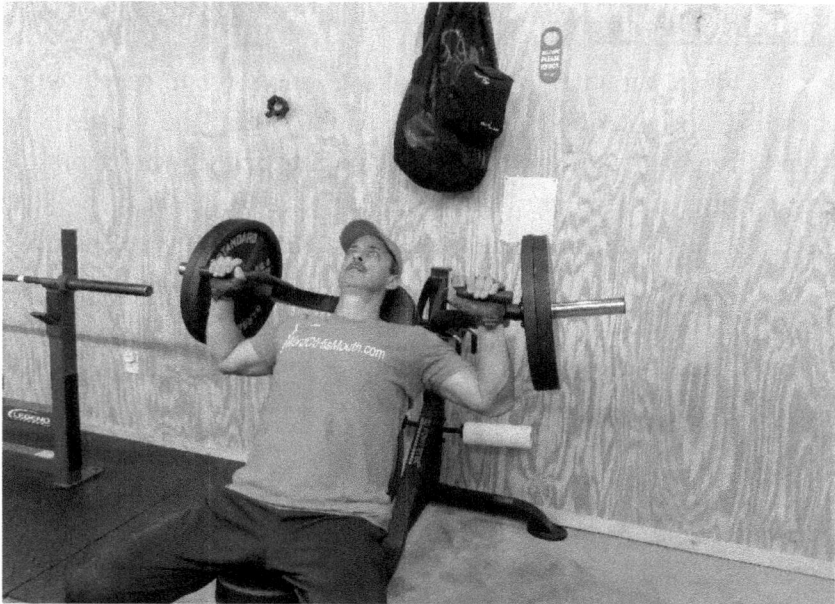

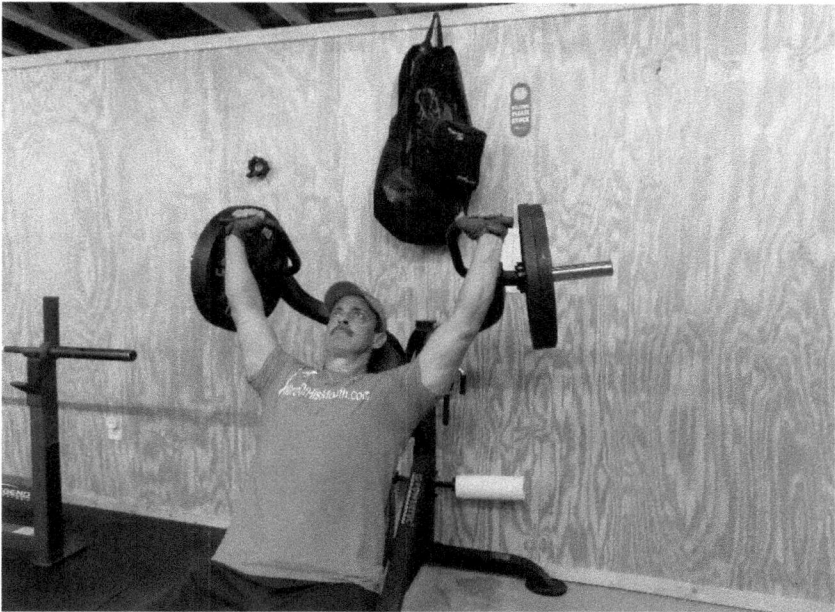

Shoulder shrug

With the bar or handles just below your reach when standing upright, bend your knees slightly, grip the weight, and stand upright. Keeping your arms straight, pull upward from the traps (shrug like saying "I don't know"), squeeze the traps for a second, then lower the weight again in a slow, controlled manner.

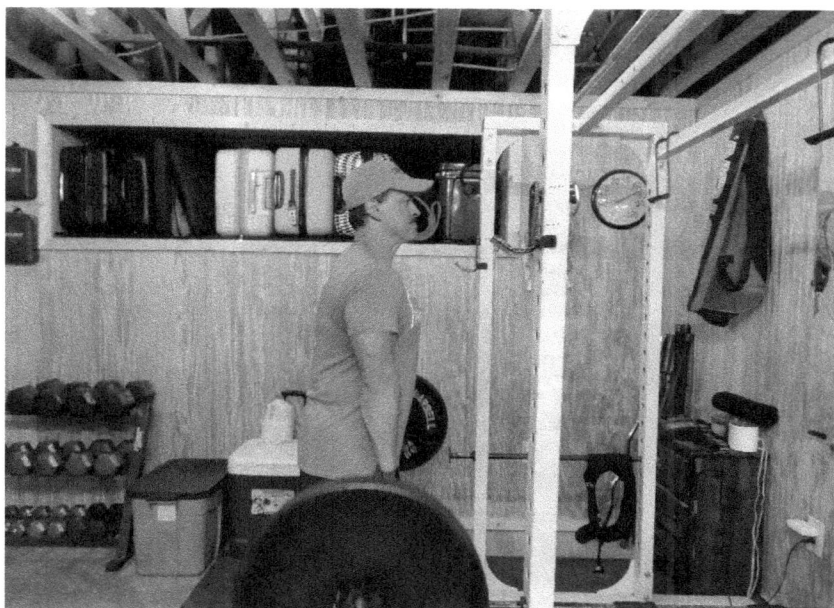

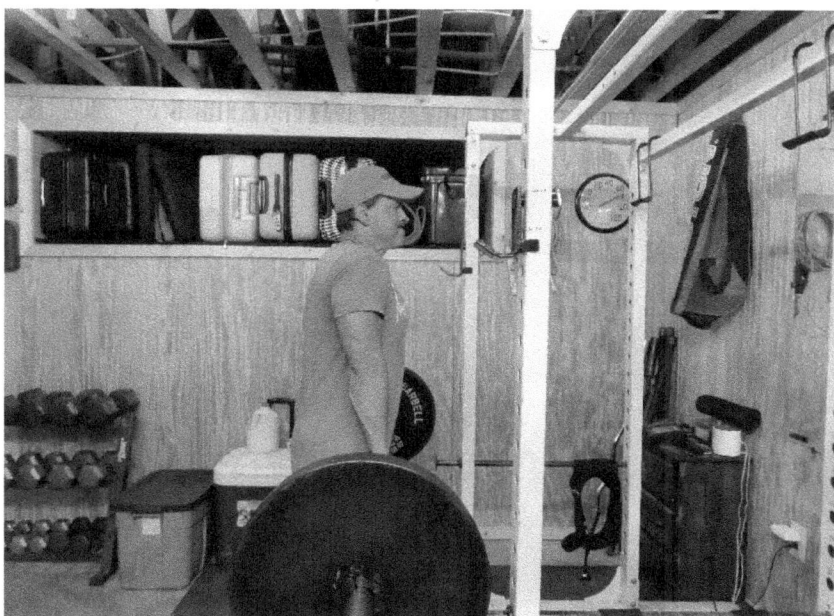

Front upward push

Using a standing calf or similar machine, put your hands under the pads in front of you and push upward. Return the weight in a slow, controlled motion.

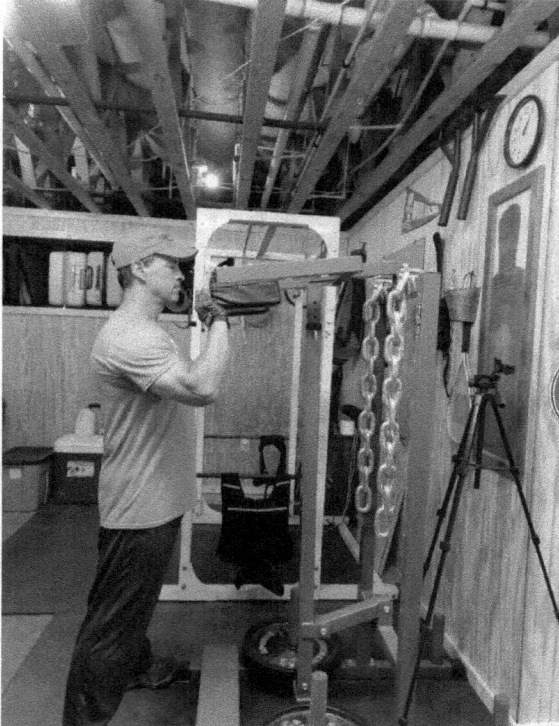

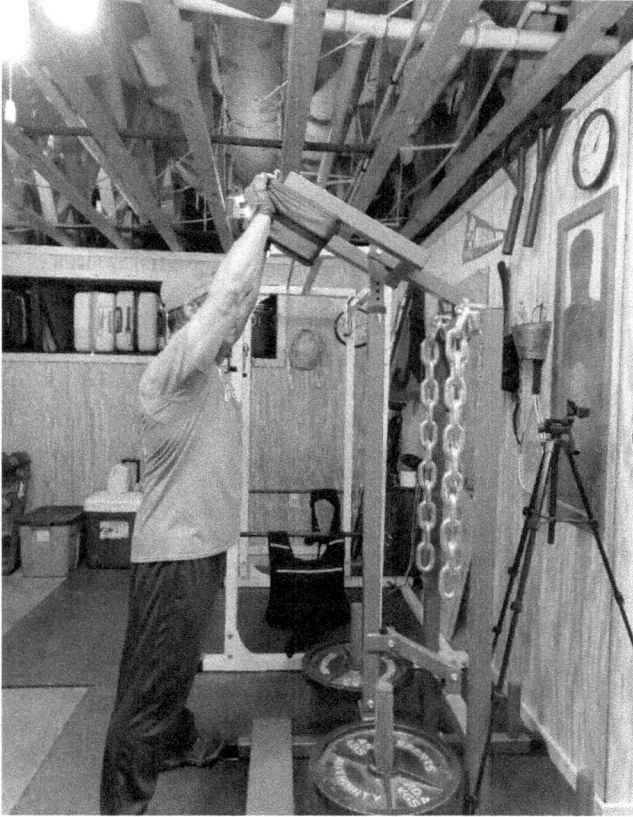

Upright barbell row

Place your hands a bit narrower than shoulder width apart. Keeping your wrists above your elbows for the entire movement, lift the bar to the level of your upper chest. Return the weight in a slow, controlled manner.

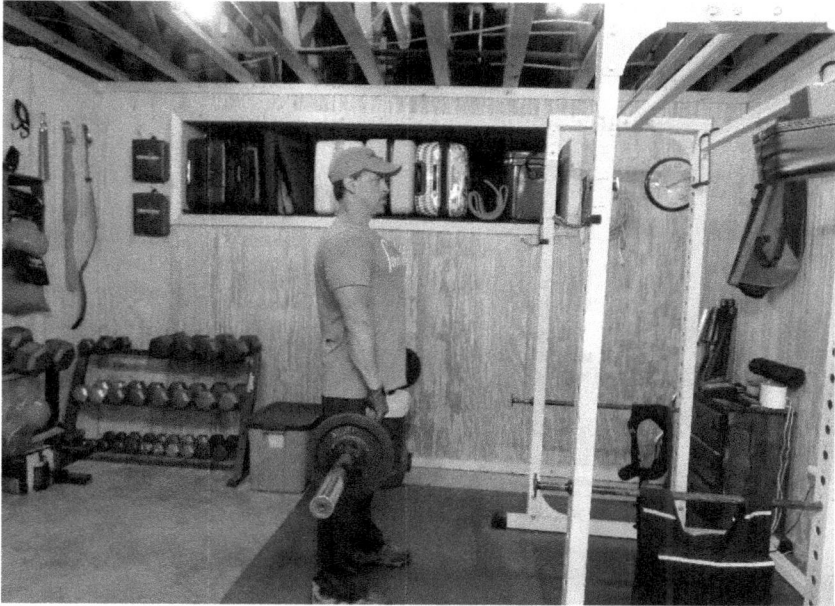

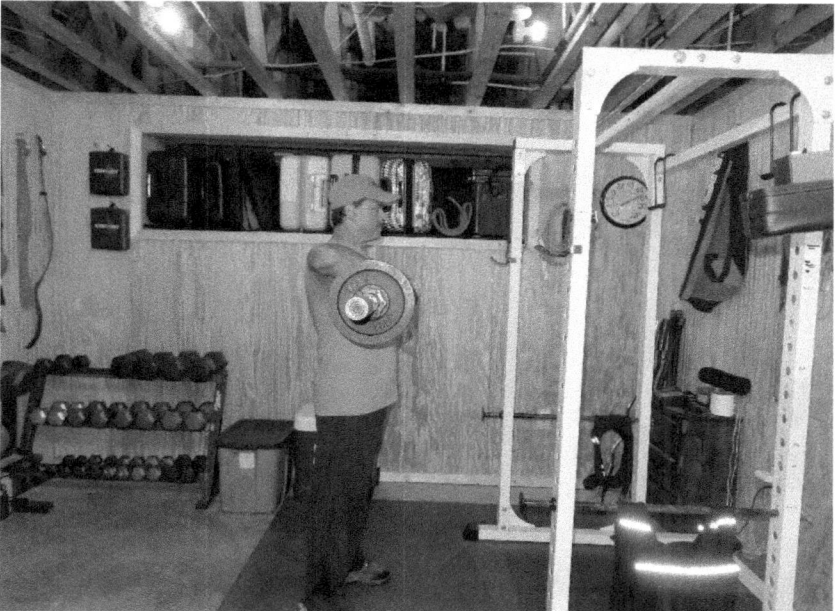

Crazy eights

With a light dumbbell in each hand, and your palms facing downward, extend both hands straight out and up eight times, then repeat at a 45-degree angle, and then repeat directly out from your sides.

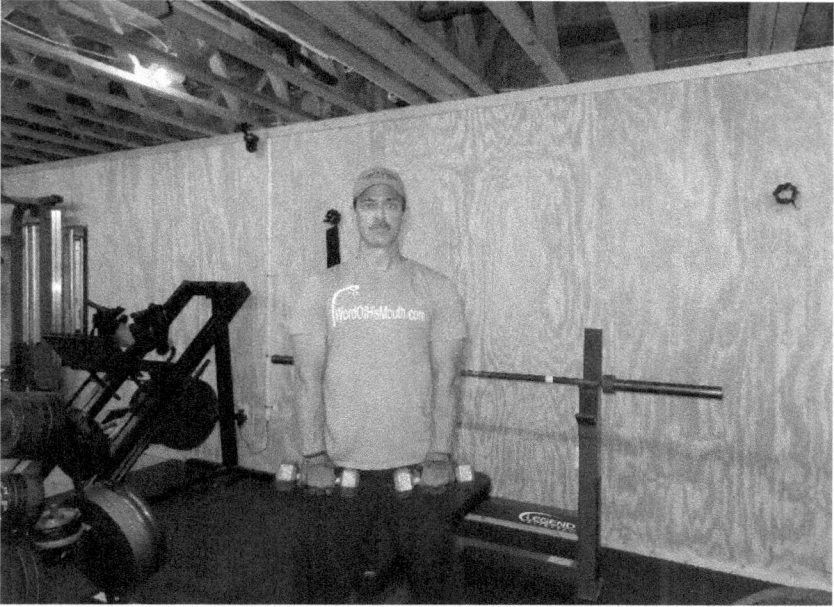

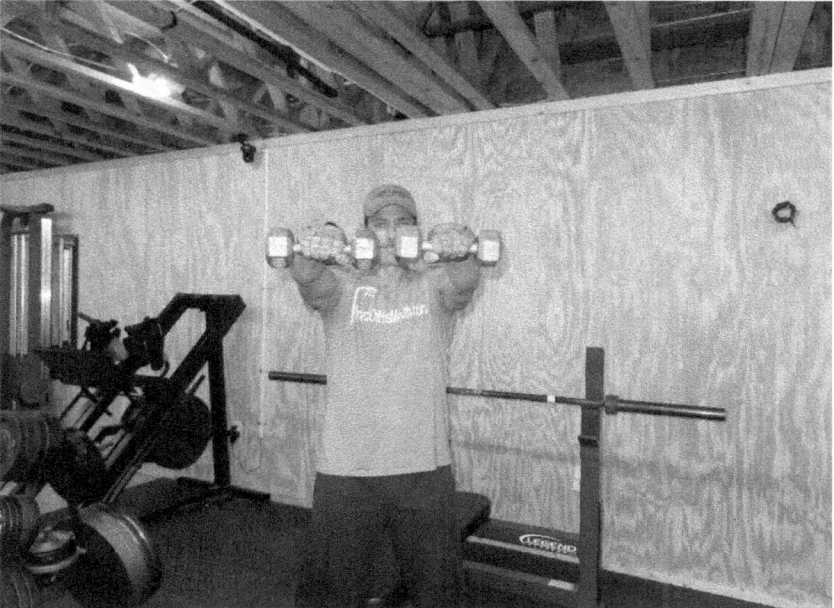

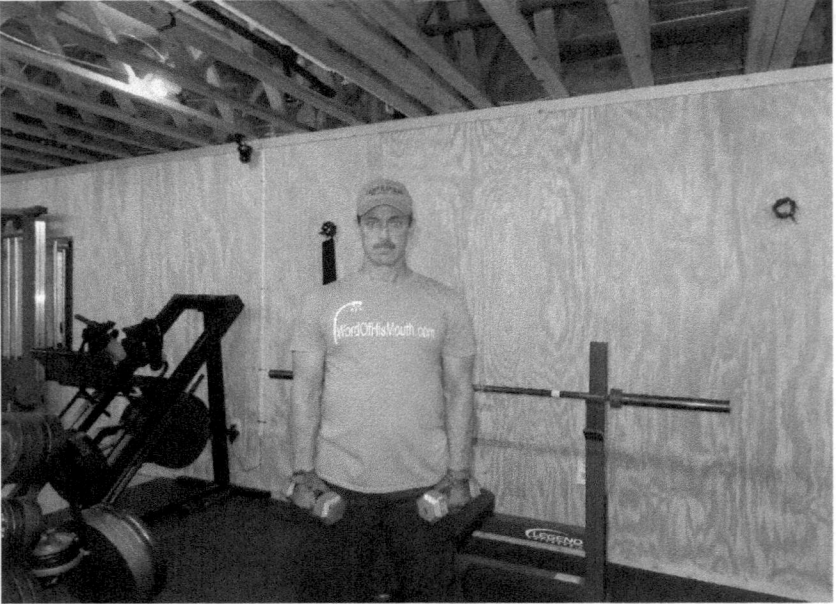

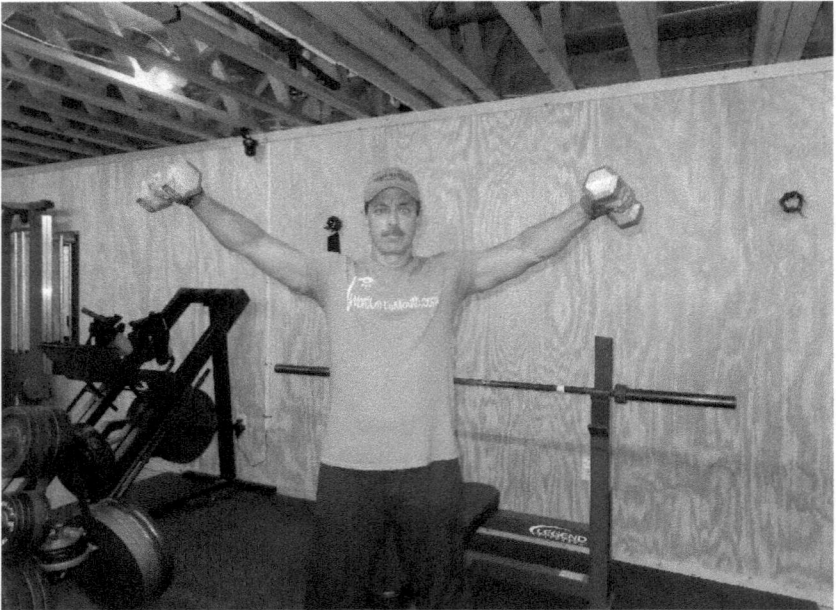

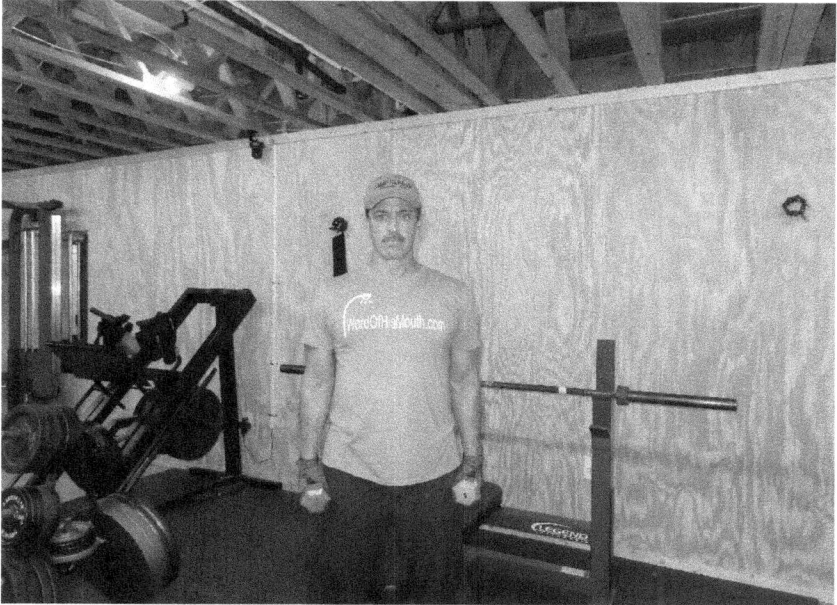

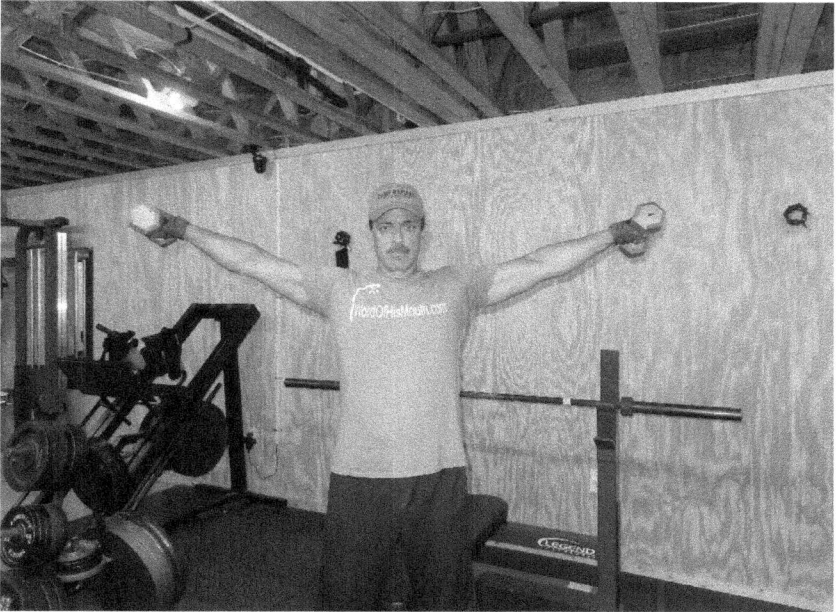

Plate shrugs

Gripping the plates directly by your side, shrug them upward, and then return the weight in a slow, controlled motion.

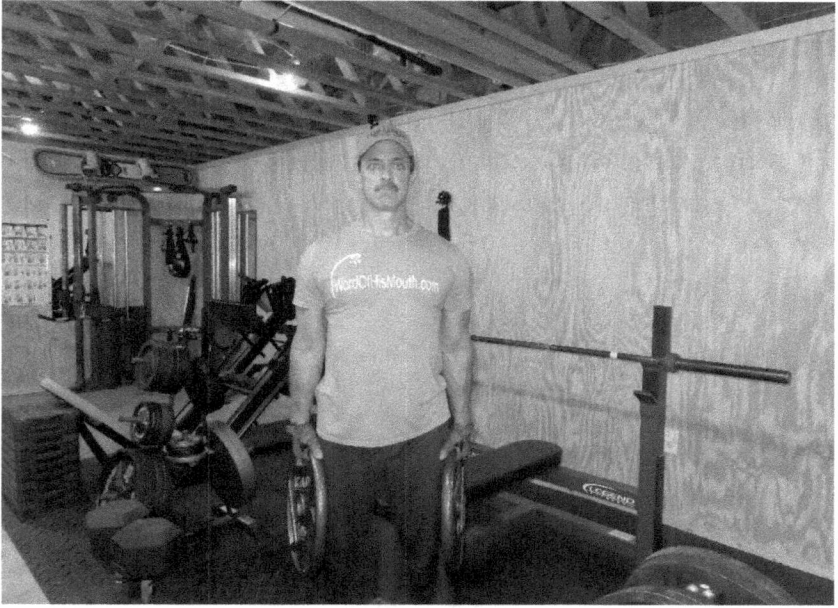

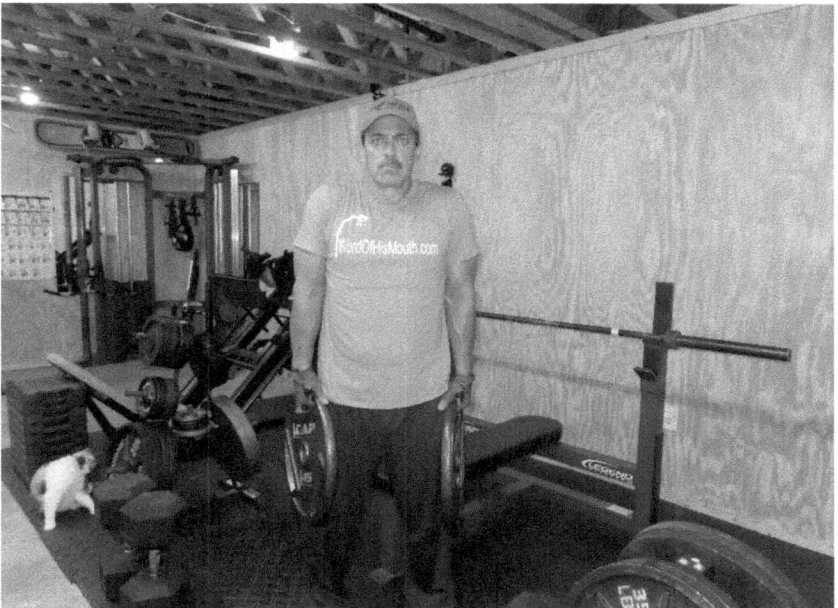

Handstand presses. *Just for fun

Either in a frame or with someone holding your legs upright, and with your hands elevated off the floor on stable platforms, push your body upward, then, in a slow, controlled manner, lower it down again.

Legs

<u>Leg press on the leg press machine</u>

Warning! **Make very sure never to lock your legs completely out** on this exercise and machine.

With your feet roughly shoulder-width apart, push the weight forward slightly, and unlock the stopping bars. Then lower the weight as far as you safely can, and push it back up into place, without completely locking your knees out at the top.

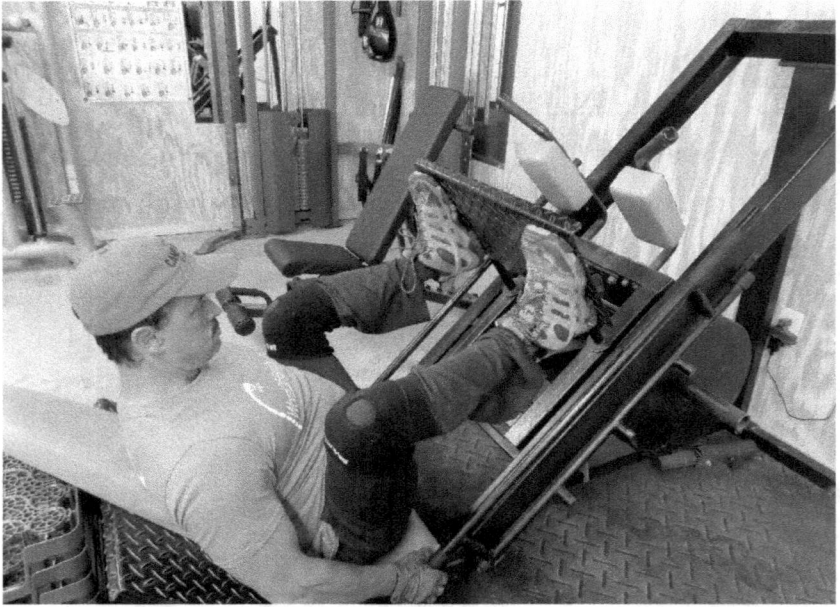

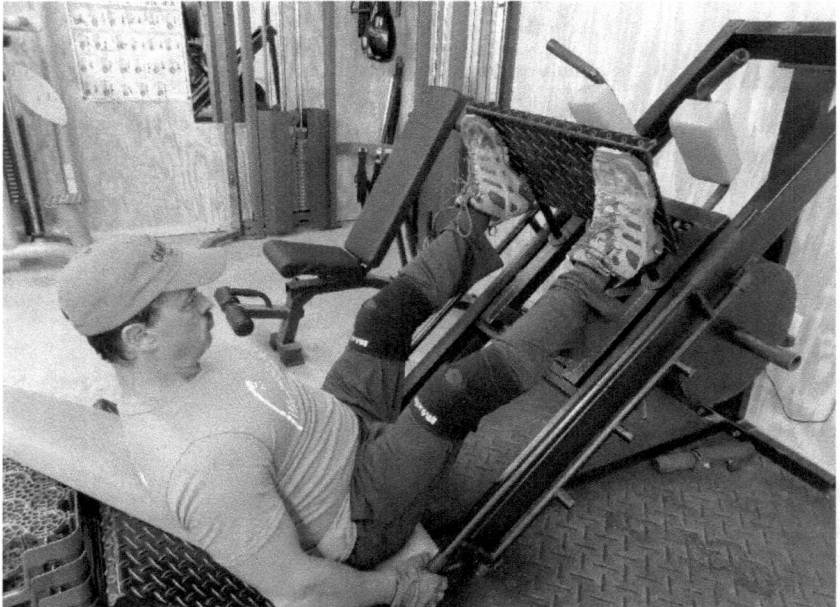

Hack squat

With your feet roughly shoulder-width apart and your shoulders underneath the pads, push upward with your legs and unlock the stopping bars. Bend your knees and lower yourself and the weight as far as you can comfortably do so, then push upward back to the upright position.

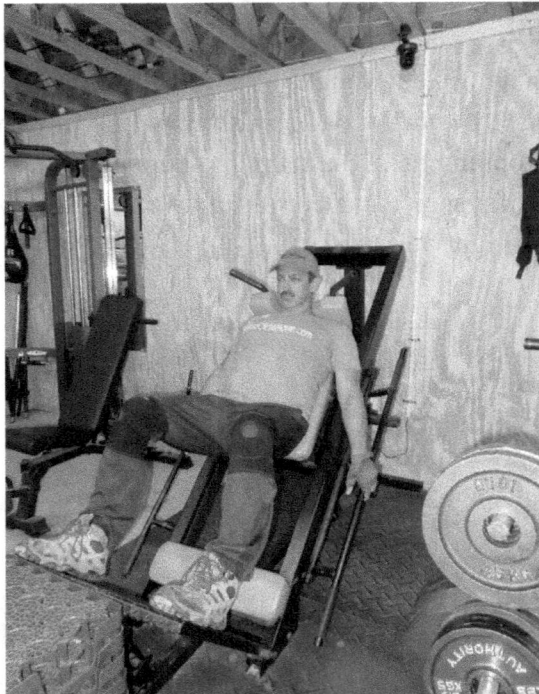
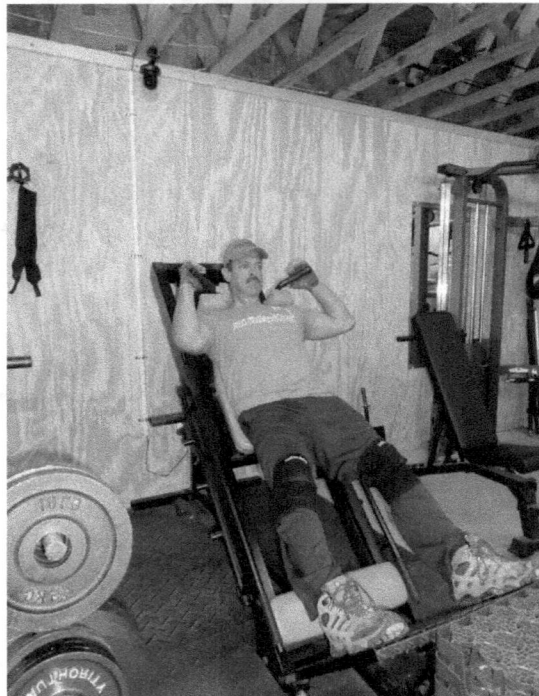

Calf Raise on Leg Press

Place your feet not too far apart from each other, and in the center of the push plate, with only the toes and balls of your feet contacting the metal. Then, with the machine locks still in place, simply pivot your feet forward, as if standing up on your tiptoes. Then lower the weight down again.

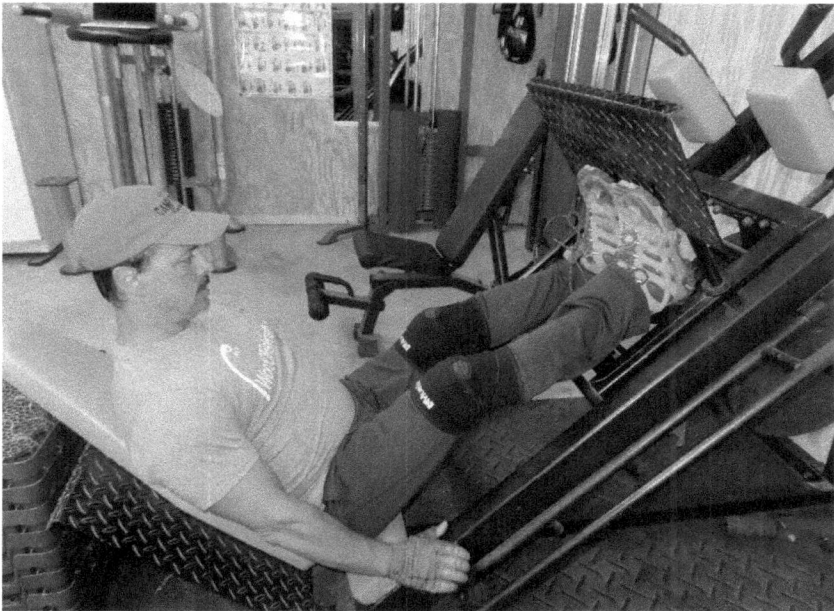

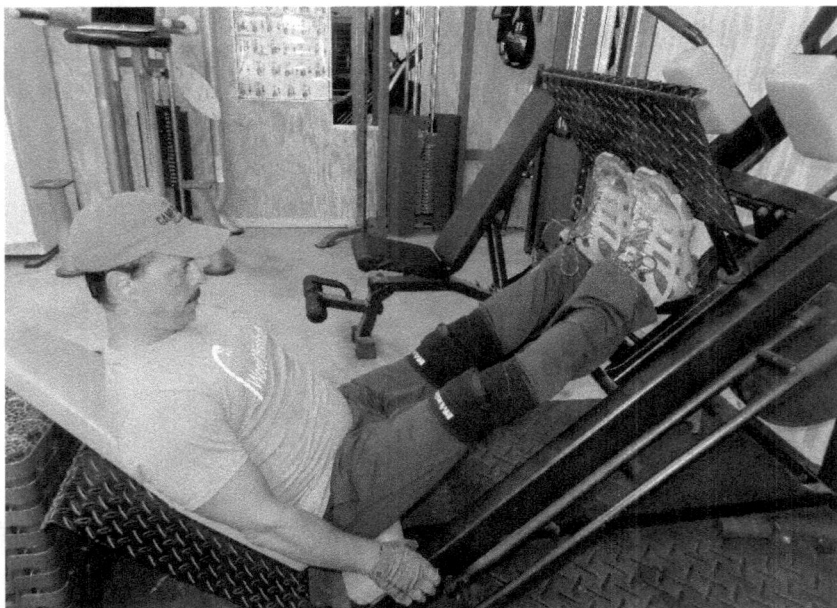

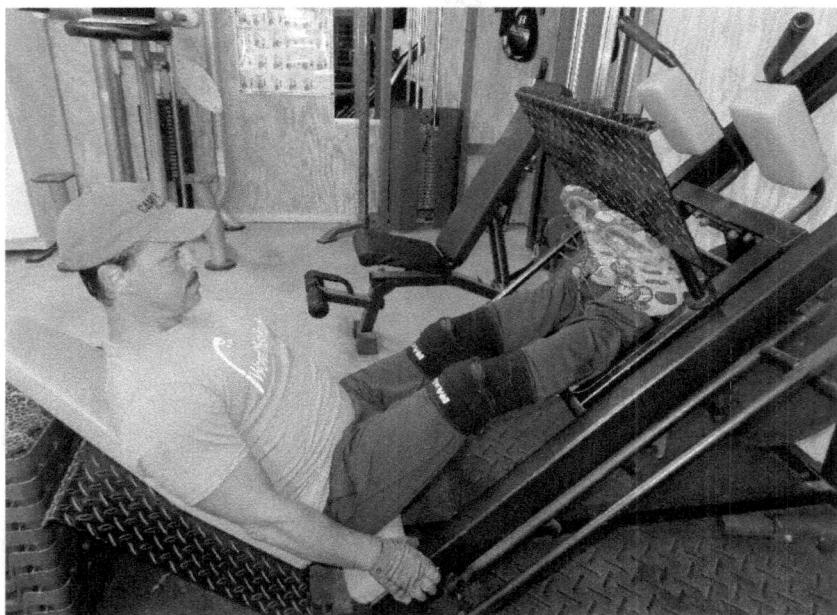

Standing calf machine

With the balls and toes of your feet on the platform, push upwards to stand on your tiptoes, pausing briefly at the very top of the movement. Then lower yourself down again in a slow, controlled manner.

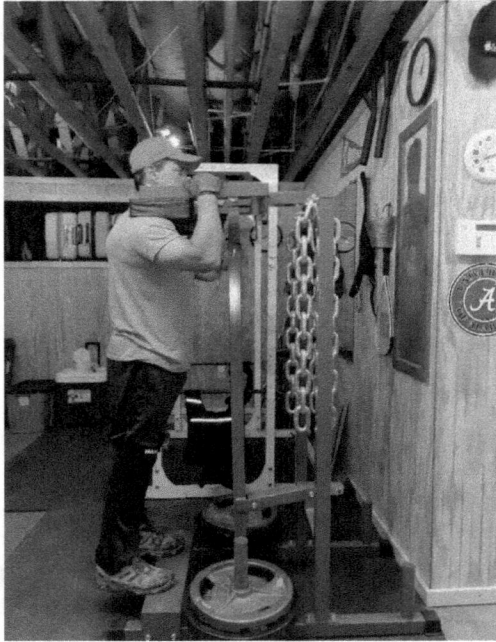

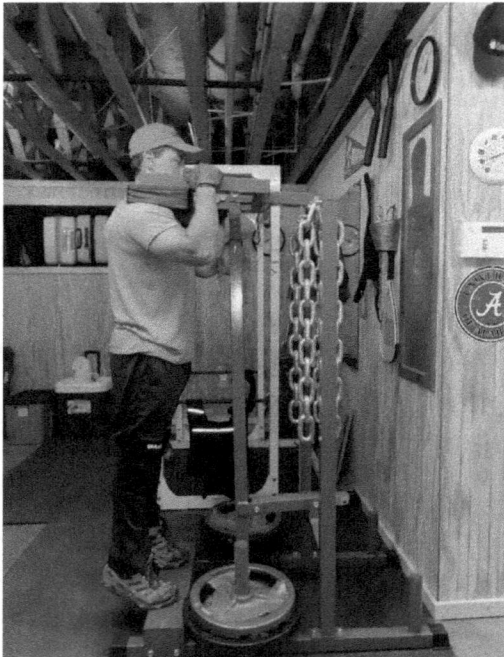

Leg extension

With your legs and feet in the proper position, extend your legs outward from the knee, pausing briefly at full extension, and then lower the weight back to the starting position in a slow, controlled manner.

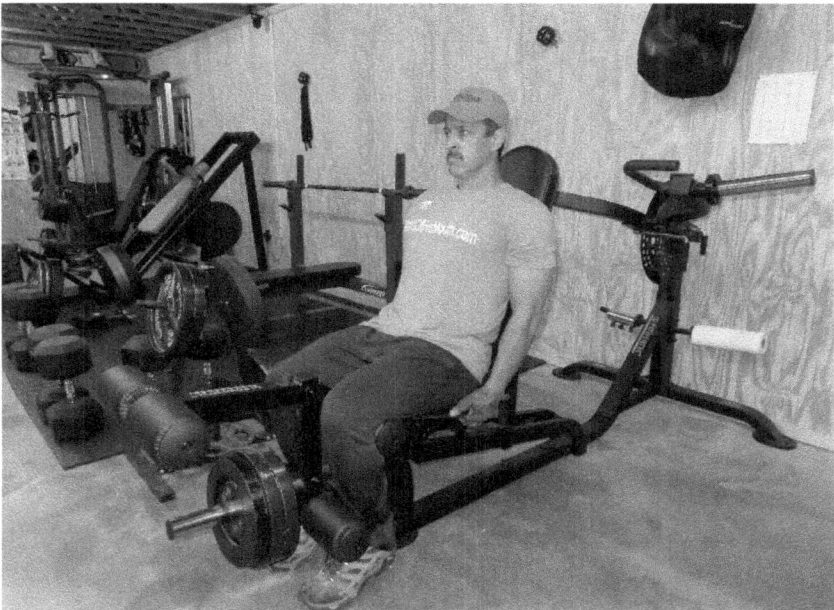

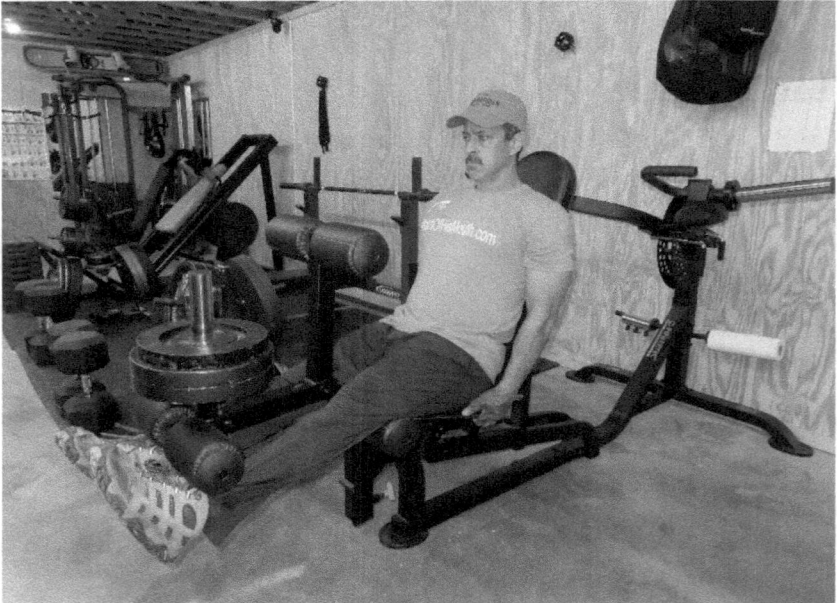

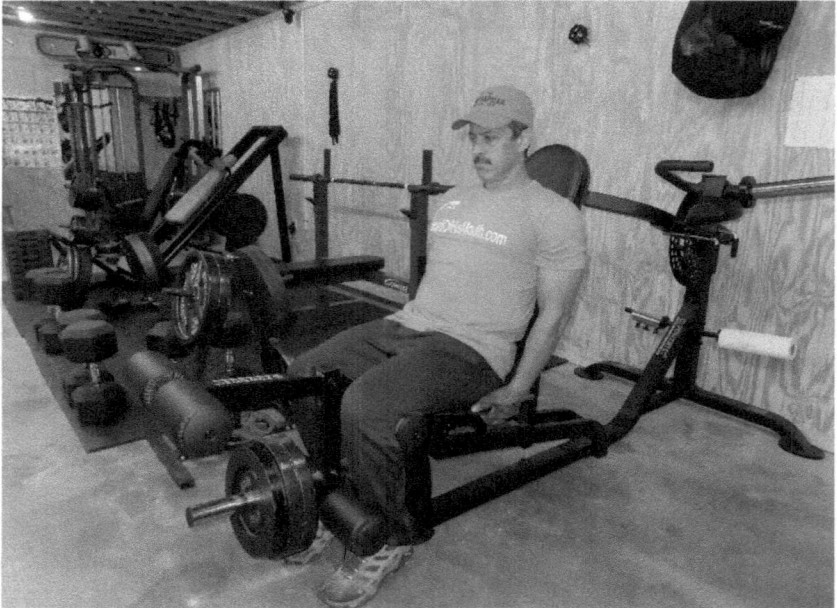

Leg curls

Lying face down on the machine, grip either the sides of the pad or whatever bars are provided to hold, and curl your legs and the weight upward from the knees, pausing briefly at full contraction. Then lower the weight back to the starting position in a slow, controlled manner.

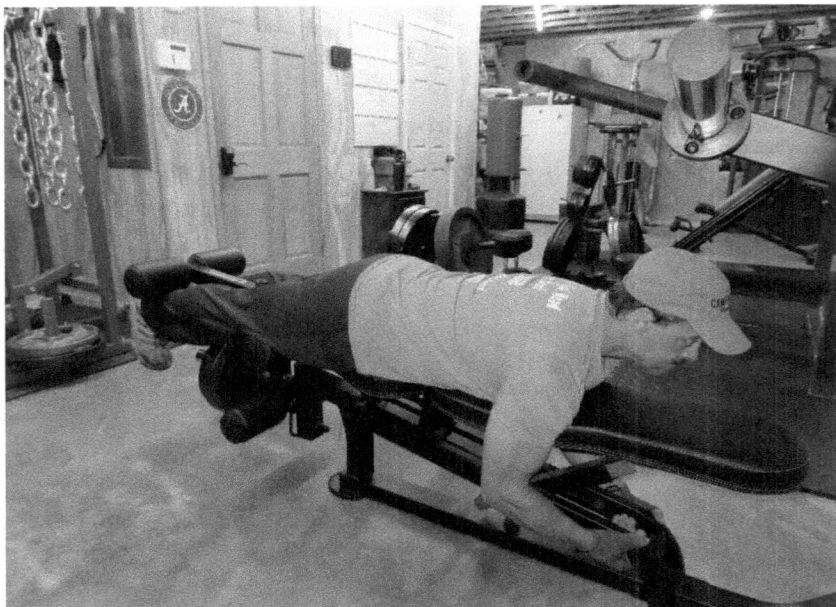

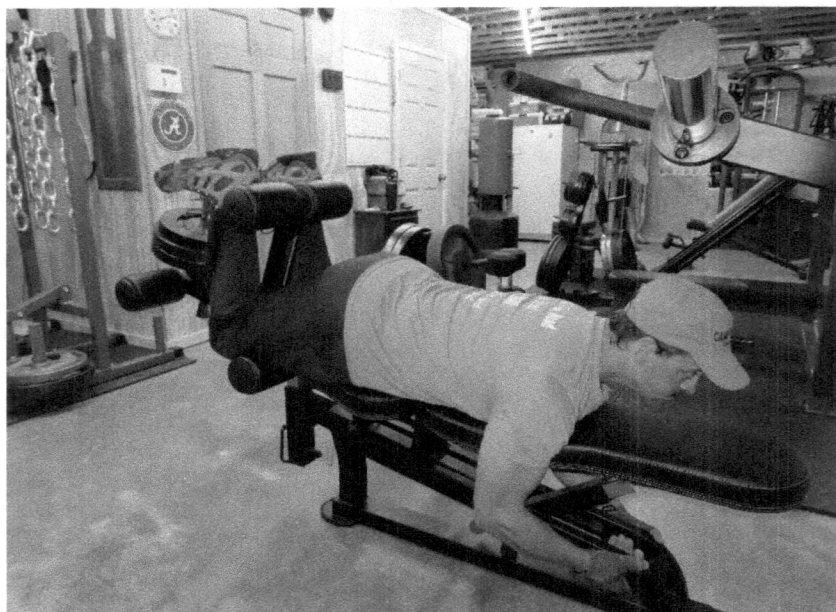

Core exercises

<u>Crunches</u>

With your legs either up on a prop or suspended in air, put your hands beside your head. Do not lock them behind your head, or you will invariably try to pull yourself upward from the neck. Focus on using your stomach muscles to curl your upper body up toward your legs, then lower yourself down again, maintaining tension on the abs the entire time.

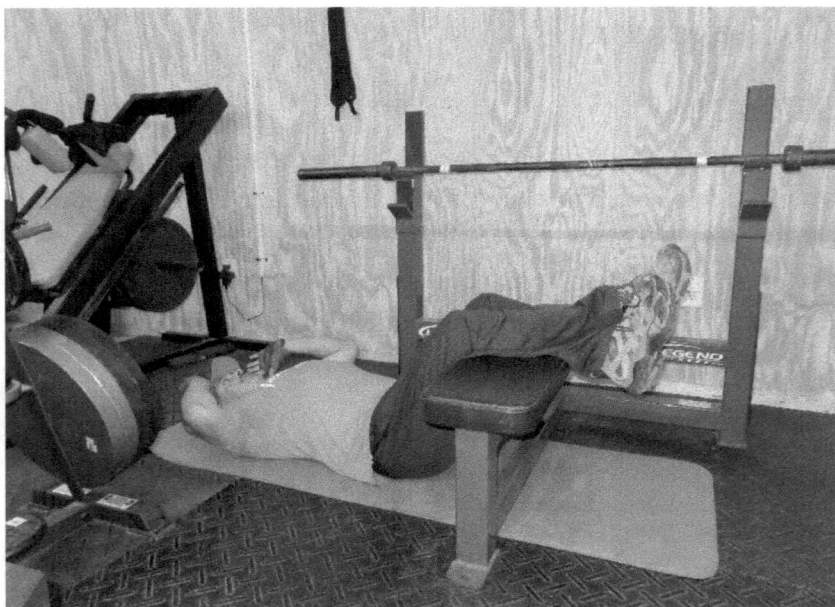

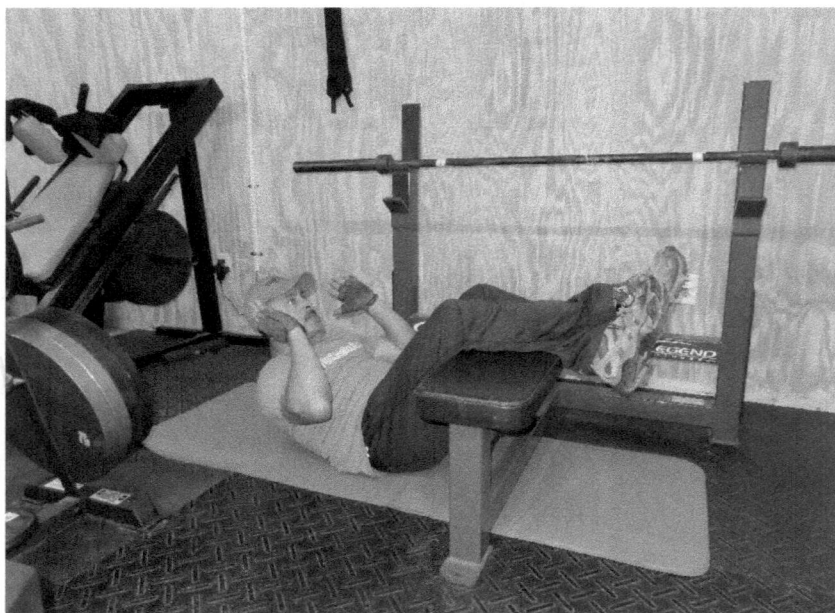

Flutter kicks

Lying on your back with your legs straight out in front of you, put your hands close beside and even a bit underneath your bottom. Then elevate your legs several inches off the floor, kick one upward while bringing the other down over and over again. At the same time, pull your torso upward slightly to add to the tension on your abs.

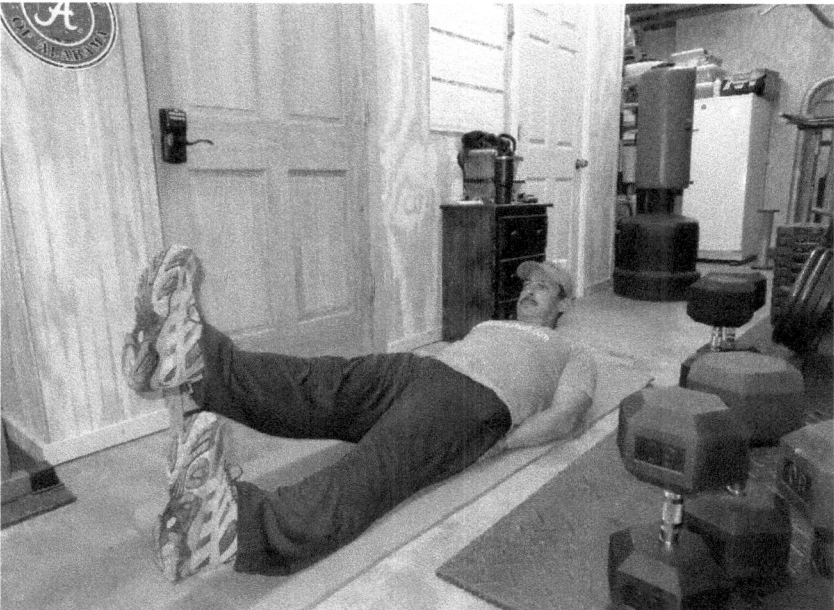

Reverse Crunches

Lying flat on your back with your arms either beside you or slightly spread out and your legs on the ground straight in front of you, pull your knees to your chest, then lower them down again.

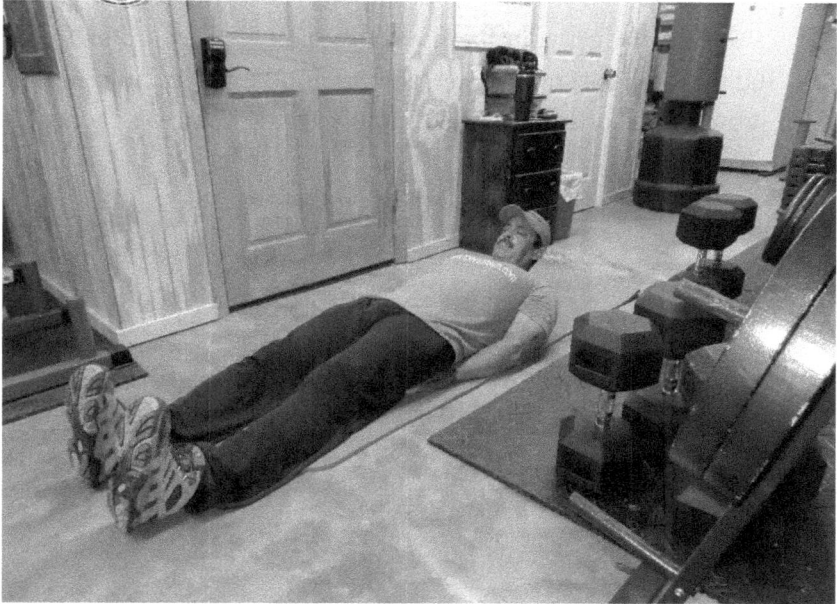

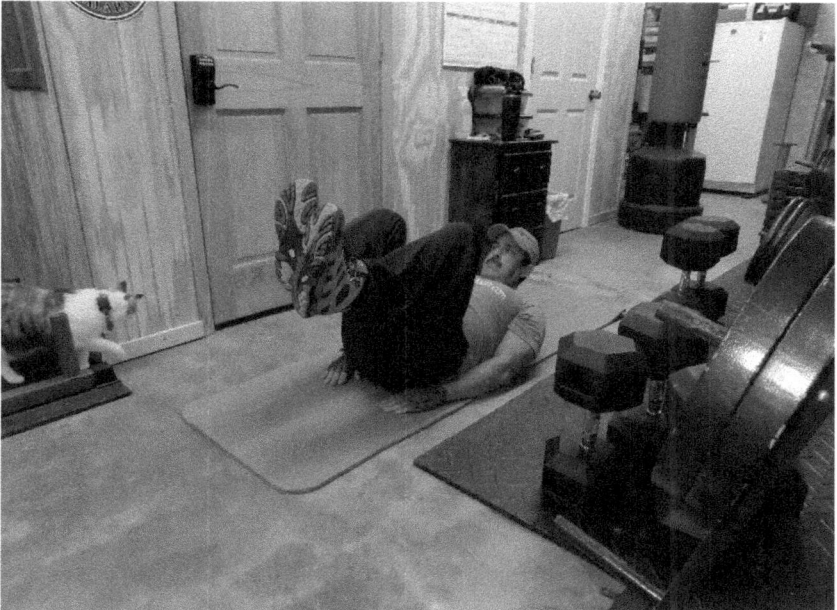

Oblique ankle taps

Lying flat on your back with your knees upward and your feet flat on the floor, raise your torso to good tension, hold it, then shift it back and forth repeatedly, tapping your ankle on each side.

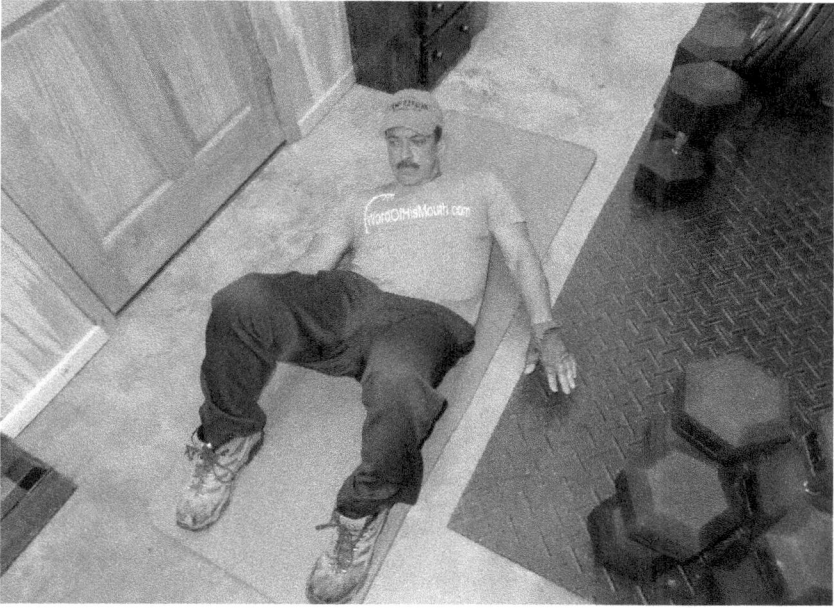

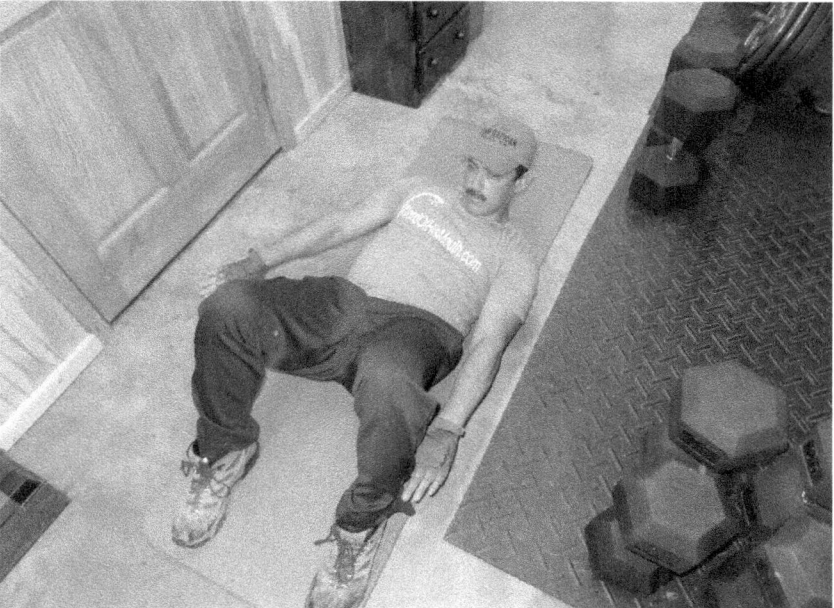

Planks

Resting on your elbows, raise your body to plank position and hold it for 30-60 seconds, then lower down again.

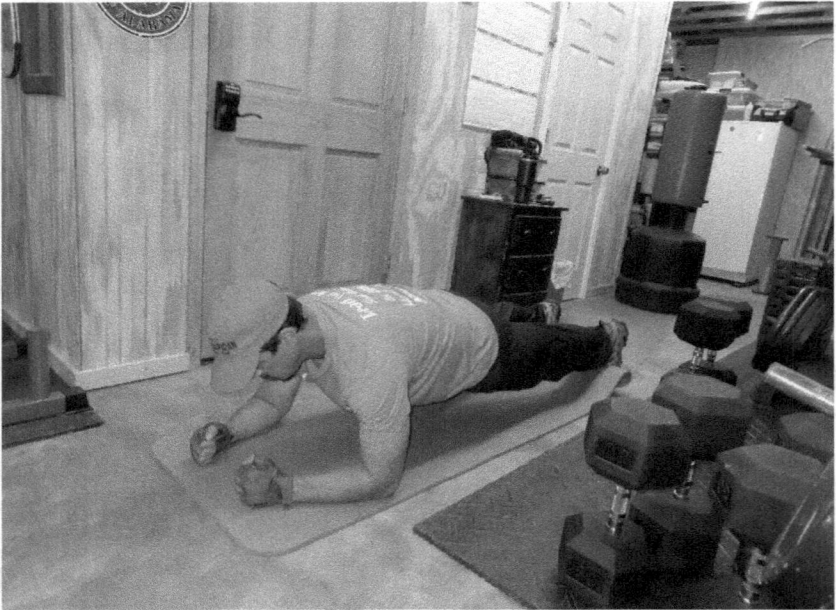

Weighted side bends

Using either a plate or a dumbbell, lean your body slightly to the side, then pull yourself back up to the starting position.

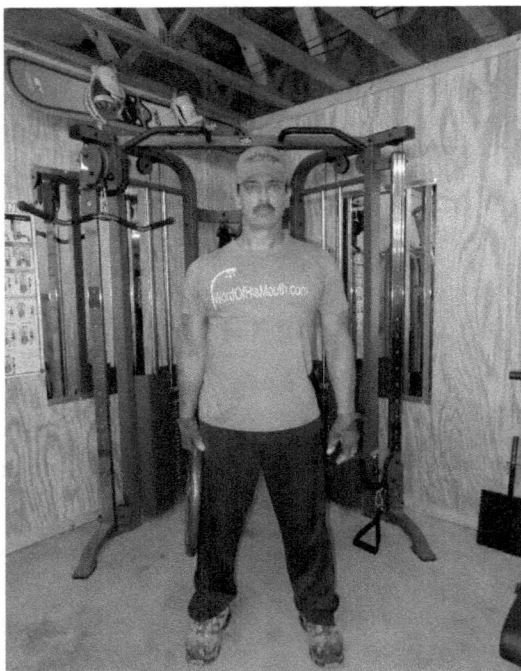

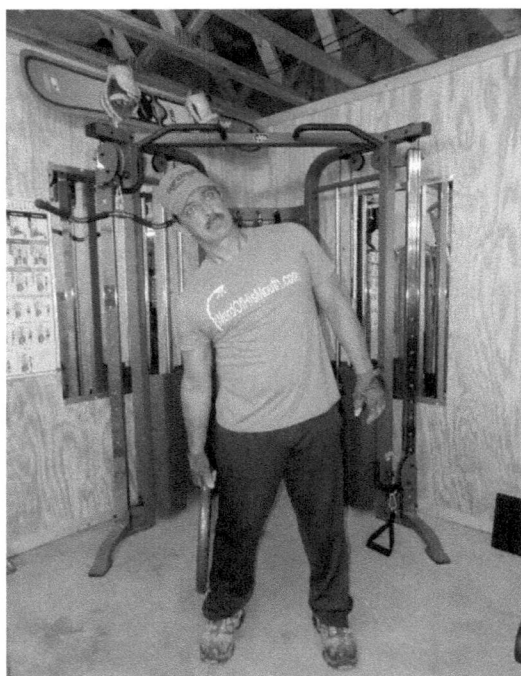

Occasional Others

Farmer's Carry

The farmer's carry is excellent for the shoulders, forearms, grip strength, and even provides a cardio boost. Simply hold a weight in each hand and take a walk with it. For an extra challenge, use stairs.

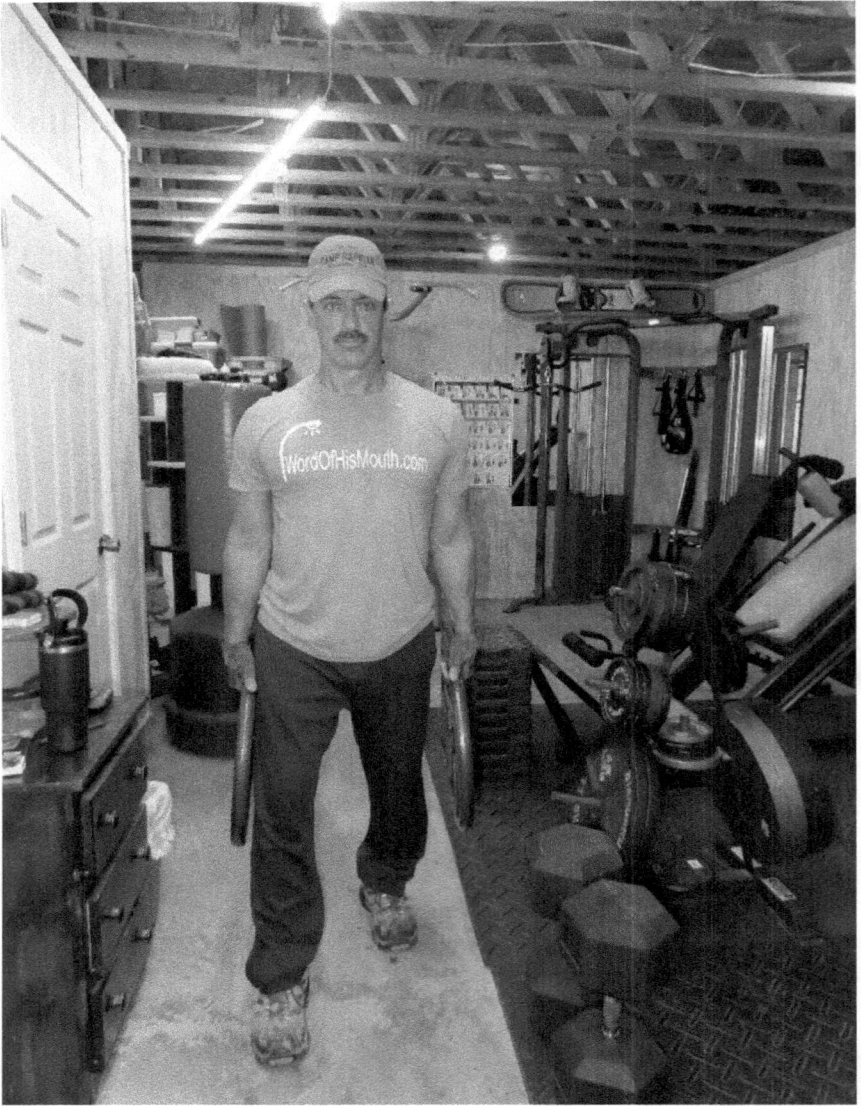

Static Holds

Static holds are excellent for the shoulders, forearms, grip strength, and back. Simply hold a weight in each hand until you have to put it down.

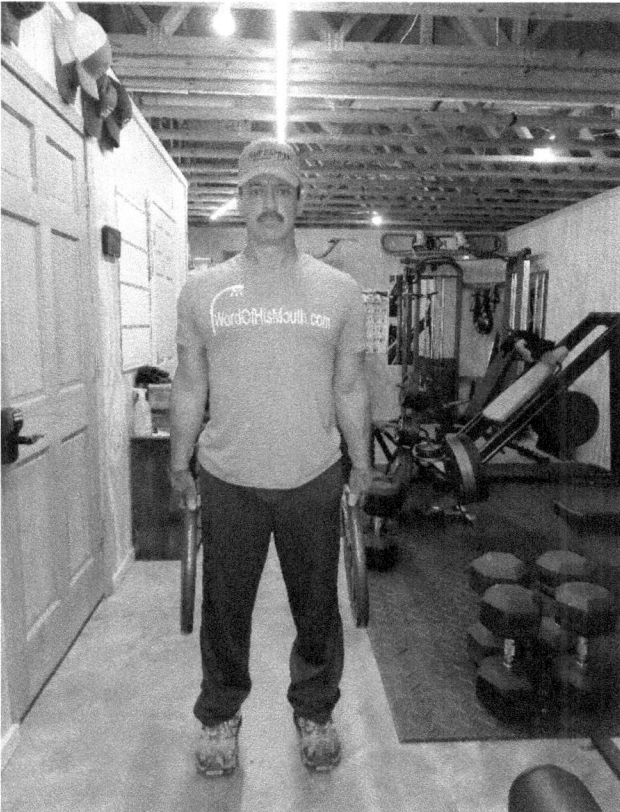

Land Mines

Using a land mine bar, brace yourself at an angle, and push upward from the shoulder.

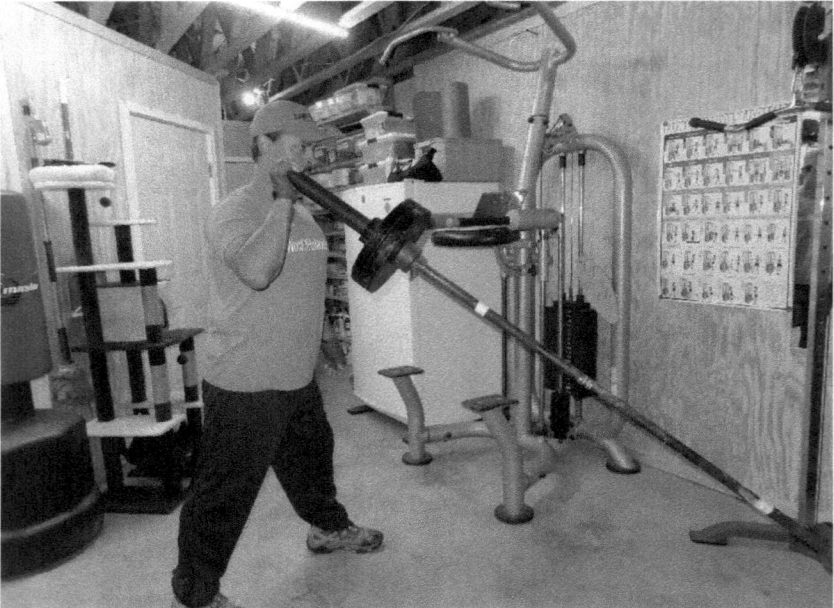

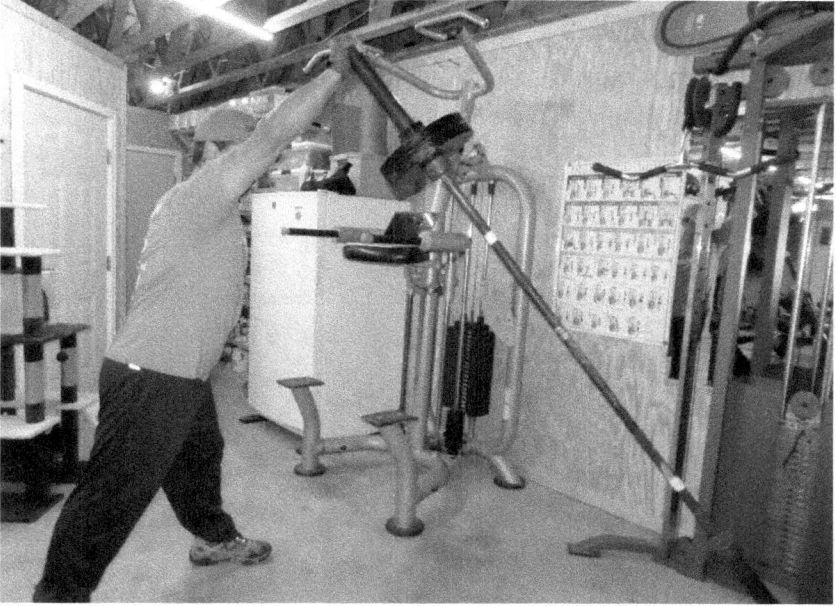

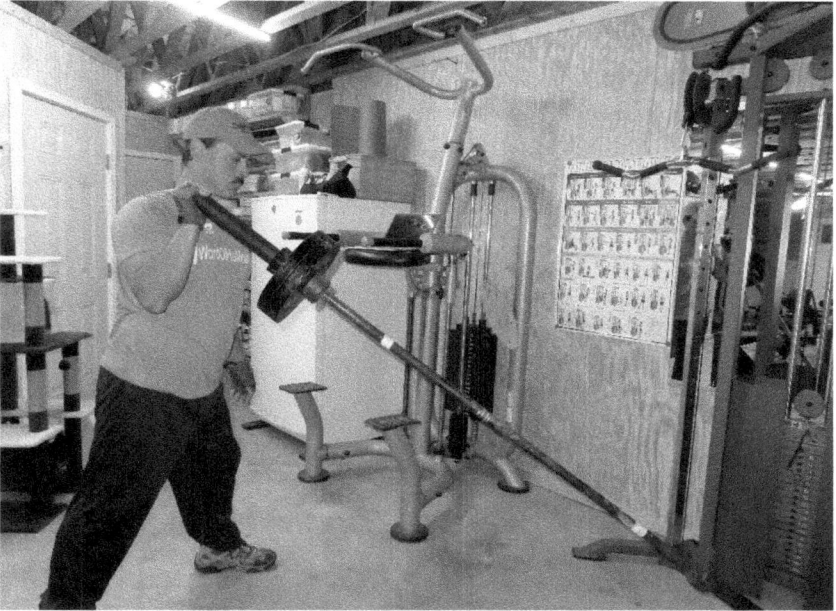

Flex Cable Curls

With a handle on either side at shoulder height, and using a light weight, curl your arms as if flexing. Hold for a second, then lower the weight again.

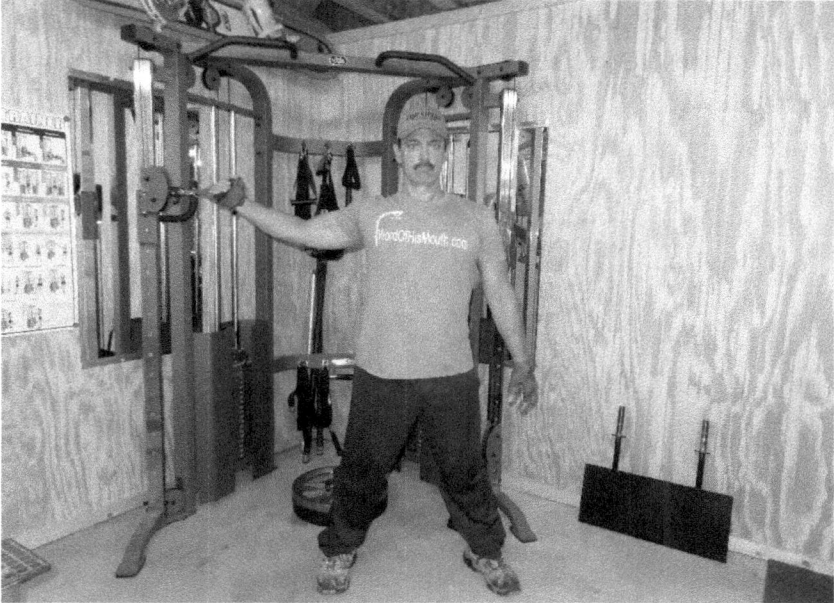

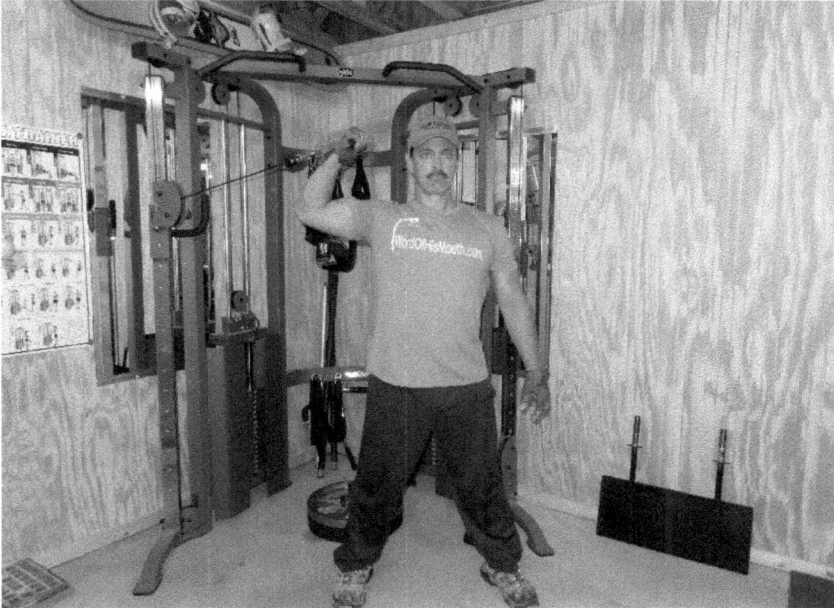

Here is a link to a video demonstrating how to perform many of these exercises using workout bands, courtesy of Pastor Chris Hewett.

Chapter Eight
Run for Your Life!

And now, dear reader, I turn you over to a dear friend, Pastor Austin Vetsrand, for a discussion on running. He is far more of an expert on this than I am, and I knew you would benefit from his perspective and insight. Bo Wagner.

We have all heard the jokes told by a person taking Scripture out of context to try and paint running as something God is not pleased with, while at the same time painting a picture that an unhealthy, lethargic, and overweight person is God's "ideal" messenger: "The wicked flee when no man pursueth…" "The liberal soul shall be made fat…" Other excuses I hear to reject overall fitness are, "We are going to die anyway," and "Skinny people die too."

I know we will die, but as the dear author of this book has said many times, "I want to be as healthy as I can, as long as I can, to do as much as I can for the Lord." While these jokes may sound cute with reasoning that is a subtle excuse to be lazy, in reality, many are doing themselves a physical and spiritual disservice by rejecting their health, and quite frankly, running is a wonderful way to improve health so that someone may serve God longer.

I have always been in good physical condition, but I honestly hated running. At 17, I joined the United States Army Infantry (11B), and running became a way of life. For nearly six years, every week of my life was packed with running. Five mile run Mondays, never strictly on flat land, with a gym workout in the afternoon, HIIT (High Intensity Interval Training) workouts on Tuesdays, which will tremendously improve your cardio, with a gym workout in the afternoon, Wednesday, three mile runs in the morning with gym workouts in the afternoon, Thursday, two mile run with a gym workout in the afternoon, and then a six mile Ruck run on Fridays in full "BATTLE RATTLE." Of course, we also had the occasional ten-mile run included with other various intense workouts.

After I left the Military, though, I stopped running for three and a half years, and my body felt it. With blood pressure rising and heart health lowering because of a bad diet and no running, I knew I needed to make a change quickly. So I went back to running, and I immediately saw improvement. For over four years now, I have been back on my running schedule, and I feel better than ever. Knocking on doors, preaching in the pulpit and on the streets, the hectic schedule of pastoring and all the activities that come with the ministry have become less demanding physically with regular running.

There are numerous benefits to running. Running specifically targets the cardiovascular system. This is the portion of your body that circulates blood in your body and includes the heart, blood, and blood vessels. The stronger your cardiovascular system, the stronger your heart pumps, the lower your heart rate, the lower your blood pressure, the lower your cholesterol, the greater your lung capacity, and the more unrestricted your blood flows. Having a resting heart rate of 85 is not good; running will get that down. Having blood pressure running 155/93 is not good; running will get that down. Running leads to an increase in VO2 max, and the higher this max, the better your body will be at utilizing the oxygen in your body. The higher this max, the more you will be able to sustain activity that works your heart.

Running lowers stress while releasing intense amounts of dopamine, relaxing the mind and body (and honestly, stress will kill you quicker than anything). These benefits will make you more effective as a Christian. You will be able to be of more service to Christ when you have less stress, great cardiovascular health, and fewer hospital stays. What testimony do we show when we cannot even knock on doors for an hour? At the same time, I am not naïve, and I understand that people sometimes have health issues beyond their control because of injuries, genetics, etc., that affect different aspects of their health. But we should not compound our health problems when we already have them because of these issues by refusing to exercise our bodies. It is difficult for folks with leg and hip issues to run, but I am thankful there are other options that are easier on the body (we will look at those later).

Proper nutrition is very important when considering the long-term benefits of running. While thinking that having a triple bypass, seven heart stents, and comparing cholesterol medicine with friends is somehow "spiritual," many Christians neglect good and healthy foods in favor of foods that will put them in the grave early (Ecclesiastes 7:17).

I am not against pizza, donuts, etc., and as a matter of fact, I love those foods. But as with anything, they must be taken in moderation. I have seen too many people making jokes about nutrition and exercise, take five steps out knocking on doors, and then not even able to catch their breath because their arteries are clogged with calcium from too many Baconators. We all hear it now, the "super Christian" quotes, out of context again, such as 1 Timothy 4:4-5, "For every creature of God is good, and nothing to be refused, if it be received with thanksgiving: For it is sanctified by the word of God and prayer."

My answer is this: I contest whether anything coming from a fast food joint is a "creature" of God rather a creation of man in a lab! I always laugh to myself when I hear people preach on smoking cigarettes and then go eat a double quarter pounder with cheese, which clogs arteries and stops hearts at a much faster rate. (Studies show that 11 million people die worldwide a year from bad diets, while 8 million die from the effects of smoking.)

Eat foods in moderation. Many people think dieting is the way to good health, but this is not true. Our eating habits must be a way of life, not a "diet." What you eat will directly impact how

173

well you run, and unhealthy foods that hurt heart health will impede your ability to run. Drinking plenty of water and eating plenty of veggies (especially greens), fruits and nuts (walnuts and almonds especially), fish (haddock and salmon are great choices), whole and sprouted grains, lean chicken, and healthy beans are all great foods that will help you in your running journey.

Getting started in running is not difficult. Most importantly, it takes DISCIPLINE. Without personal accountability and discipline, you will never last as a runner. Running can be the most mundane task you do, especially if you live in an area with dull scenery. Get a good pair of running shoes because your feet will be your most important asset (Asic, Hoka, and Brooks are great brands for running shoes, with each having different varieties for trail running, marathon running, and short-distance speed running). Make sure stretching is a vital part of your running regimen; otherwise, you will have many off days nursing a pulled hammy, thigh, calf, or groin.

Stretching before your run and after your run on your cool down is vital, so make sure stretches that target the feet, calves, hamstrings, thighs, groin, back, and hips are at the forefront of your mind. Make sure your running form is correct. Have a good posture, relaxed arms and shoulders, and have a quick cadence with your feet. Pounding all your body weight on pavement is a quick way for knee pain, shin splints, and Achilles pain.

Hydration is of the utmost importance. Make sure you are drinking plenty of water and use electrolytes in water (stay away from sugary and caffeinated drinks). I drank over a gallon of water a day in the Army and drink nearly a gallon now. Start off with short, slow runs and work your way up in mileage. Starting with a one-mile run at a slow pace for a beginner is a good start. Gradually work up the mileage to build endurance in your muscles while simultaneously increasing your pace (for example, I can run four miles in 28:48. This takes time to build up to, but with perseverance, it will come). Marathon runners typically train four months leading up to their race, increasing distance and intensity, eventually up to 26.2 miles. Short-distance speed runners focus more on HIIT workouts, crossover workouts, and interval runs that build speed for bursts within a five-mile distance.

As mentioned earlier, I understand not everyone can physically run. Maybe you were in a bad car accident and it permanently damaged your hips. Maybe you have had knee replacements, and it impedes your ability to run. Whatever the case may be, there are alternative options to running that improve your cardio. Stationary bikes, row machines, swimming, and jumping rope are all great ways to improve cardio. One of the most effective ways to improve cardio is just taking a good, old-fashioned walk. Walking is easy on the joints but very good for the heart. I encourage you to do whatever you can to get out and stay active and control what you can control with your heart health. Are there health issues out of our control? Yes, but if we do what we can, we will be a good steward with the heart God has given us and be able to use it for God's glory.

The goal is not to make a god out of fitness, but to use it as a tool to be in tip-top shape as a soldier in the Lord's army. The work of the Lord is demanding on our bodies; long days and late nights in spiritual warfare wear us down, compress our hearts, and make it easy for us to adopt an unhealthy lifestyle, which I believe Satan uses to get us out of the fight. Many preachers, especially, have been taken out of the fight early because of physical issues that were within their realm of control; let us not be guilty of this!

Best wishes on your running journey!

Austin Vetsrand

Chapter Nine
Rules of the Gym

When you see the words "Rules of the gym," you likely have in mind something that we weightlifters call "gym etiquette." And while I am all in favor of gym etiquette and aware of the fact that in certain cases it can be dangerous not to exercise gym etiquette, especially in settings where it is evident that you are among crazed, juiced up lunatics who are very particular about "their stuff," that is not what I have in mind by these words for this title.

What I do have in mind are certain principles of exercise and health that I have developed through the years. Think of them as sort of my version of the "Gym 10 Commandments." These are guidelines that I have found very helpful to keep me motivated. And this is pretty important, because I can assure you that most of the people who start an exercise program do not last very long. In fact, they usually last up until that initial burst of motivation goes away.

These, then, are some principles that will hopefully keep you going until you see your goals achieved.

Rule number one: If you can't do everything, do one thing.

Each of my full workouts ranges anywhere from forty-five minutes to an hour and forty-five minutes. But the funny thing about life is that it does not always cooperate with our schedule. Especially in ministry, everything from hospital visits, to funerals, to weddings, to counseling, to special meetings, to plumbing problems, to a broken-down church van, to a pressing assignment, and a million things more can intrude on any given day. And this means that forty-five minutes to an hour and forty-five minutes, especially at some prime time of the day, is not always possible to come by. What is generally left, then, is a few moments at a less-than-optimal time in which you have a choice to make: do I do nothing since my regular time and plans have been scuttled? Or do I do something even if it cannot possibly be a full workout?

If you can't do everything, do one thing.

As I discussed earlier, there are many days that I find myself going into the gym relatively late at night to do ten or fifteen minutes worth of just one exercise. Can I get a full workout in with that period of time? Certainly not. But what I can do is keep my muscles active and engaged, and keep myself in the habit of going to the gym. It's sort of like going to church; once you get out, it is easy to stay out, but if you stay in, it is easy to be there the next day, and the next, and the next.

Rule number two: A bad workout is better than no workout.

Full disclosure: if something is important to me, I get obsessive about it. I want every word of my messages to be perfect. I want to take fantastic care of my family. I want my workouts to be spectacular. But the drawback to that is pretty easy to see: I get very down on myself when I feel like I have not done a good job. And in working out, that mentality can be extremely counterproductive, because you will often choose not to work out if you are "not feeling it lately" or if your last workout or two have not met your expectations. But here is what you need to know: your muscles do not care about your feelings. All they care about is Time Under Tension. If they are getting that, they and you are going to benefit.

Rule number three: Moving weight is not the goal; properly engaging your muscles is the goal.

The weight on the barbell would have been hard for many people to even bench press. How, I wondered, was this non-monstrous dude planning on curling it, as he clearly intended?

As it turns out, the answer is "by swaying like a tall building during the world's worst earthquake." He rocked that puppy and himself back and forth like he was some demented gym-crackhead and "uggghhhhd!" it up into place.

And accomplished absolutely nothing, outside of a possible hernia or slipped disk.

You are going to spend a very small portion of your life in the gym; you will spend the bulk of your life elsewhere. No one cares, I repeat, no one cares that you "moved big weights." They do care when they look at you and see big, well-defined muscles. And those do not come from "moving big weights," they come from *properly engaging your muscles.* Simply put, you will become far stronger, fitter, and more functional by using the highest weight you can correctly use than you will by incorrectly lifting a higher weight.

Rule number four: Your only competition is you.

A caveat, here. Obviously, if you do powerlifting competitions (as I often do), you do have other people to compete against. So I am talking instead about your lifestyle of working out, not some actual competition. In that, legitimately, your only competition is you. You guys do not have to measure up to the giant guy bench pressing a house beside you, nor do ladies have to match up with the 18-year-old super athlete who bounces around the gym like a demented Energizer Bunny. Your goal should indeed be to be better than a particular person – you – the you from yesterday, last week, last month, last year. When you view it that way, you will benefit, because the old you is cheering the new you on to success, not hoping to beat you!

Rule number five: Brace up.

I am currently fifty-five years old. I have been listening to "used to be lifters" for a long time. Most all of them have a story to tell, usually a story of some blown-out joint that derailed their lifting days forever. And while that can happen to anyone, the simplest thing that could have been done in most cases to avoid it usually was not done:

Wear good braces.

For me, I usually wear elbow wraps, wrist wraps, gloves, and, when I do legs, knee braces. Largely because of that, my joints are (praise God!) still in very good shape, and I can still lift reasonably heavy.

Rule number six: When it comes to injuries, quicker stops can speed you up.

Let me explain. When lifting, there is natural soreness, and every lifter quickly becomes acquainted with it and familiar with it. In the words of the Marvel character, Dr. Strange, "Pain is an old friend."

But beyond natural soreness/pain, there is actual injury, and you will quickly learn to identify that as well. There will be times that you are lifting and you "pull something." At that point, there are only two kinds of lifters: dumb lifters and smart lifters. Dumb lifters "push on through it" and end up making the injury worse, requiring a longer (often much longer) recovery period, perhaps weeks or even months. Smart lifters stop right away and tend to the issue. Because of that, the smart lifter will likely be back in the gym pretty quickly, whereas "Meathead the Maniac" will be in a lounge chair getting fat for a good while.

Rule number seven: Write it down.

The reason most people quit working out pretty quickly is because they look in the mirror or on the scale and do not see much of anything in the way of results. The problem is, they are looking to try and see the end of the process from the beginning when they are still at the beginning of the process! And, not seeing what they want to see, they quit before they have worked hard enough to see it.

But if they could see actual progress along the way, they would likely hang in there until they get to the end of the process. And they could, if they were writing things down.

Here is what I mean. When you work out, record every detail. Record the exercise you did, record each set, record the weights, record the reps. And then the next time you work out that muscle group, try to do just a little bit better in something. Try to do a slightly higher weight. Try to do a slightly higher number of reps. Make some progress on paper, something that you can see that lets you know that you are getting stronger. Because if you are getting stronger, your muscles are getting fitter, and your body is changing, even if you cannot see it yet. And this kind of progress generally comes quickly, far more quickly than looking in the mirror and expecting to see a bodybuilder where the Stay Puft marshmallow man used to be.

Rule number eight: If you keep doing it, you can keep doing it.

One of the most eye-opening things I ever saw in the gym was many years ago when I was first getting started. A man in his mid-forties came in, and his mid-sixties father came in with him. They loaded 405 pounds up on the bench press, and I stopped what I was doing, waiting to see the young man get down under the weight and lift it. Imagine my surprise, then, when it was

"Pops," as his son called him, who lay down under the weight. Pops, with son egging him on, proceeded to rep it several times.

When they were done, I approached them and asked the man, "How can you still do that?" He smiled and replied, "I started, and I just never stopped."

It is evident that everyone gets older and becomes somewhat weaker as they do. But it is also evident that those who continue to work out maintain a level of strength and functionality that very much seems to defy their age. As Dick Van Dyke famously said, "In my 30s, I exercised to look good. In my 50s, to stay fit. In my 70s, to stay ambulatory. In my 80s, to avoid assisted living. Now, in my 90s, I'm just doing it out of pure defiance."

Rule number nine: Ask for help, and give help.

There are a lot of days in the gym that I remember very well. I remember the day I finally bench pressed 315 for the first time. When I racked the weight, I stood up and screamed in triumph; the entire gym stopped what they were doing and looked at me like I had lost my mind.

I remember the first time I won a bench press contest.

I remember the day I first leg pressed one thousand pounds.

But far exceeding those days, I remember the day that a grandmother came in with her slightly special needs grandson in his late teens to early 20s. In the middle of one of my sets, she came and asked me for help; they were having trouble figuring out one of the machines for her grandson to use. I stopped what I was doing, helped him, cheered him on, and he beamed and smiled ear to ear in triumph. For the next forty-five minutes or so, he asked about one machine after another, and I helped him with all of them.

Top-shelf experience, that.

In the gym, you will almost invariably find a bunch of very good people who are more than willing to help. So help others when they need it, and don't be afraid to ask others for help when you need it.

Rule number ten: Give God the glory.

I know, I know, this is not exactly standard fare for a workout book. But God gave every single one of us the chests we bench press with, the arms we curl with, the legs we leg press with, and on and on. And as Paul told the church at Corinth, "Whether therefore ye eat, or drink, or whatsoever ye do, do all to the glory of God." (1 Corinthians 10:31). What you glorify God with, God tends to bless. And I don't know about you, but I would very much like for Him to bless my waist as well as my wallet, my core as well as my church, and my shoulders as well as my service!

Chapter Ten
The Benefit of Subgroups

With the six-day workout routine, there is good news, and there is bad news. The good news is, in a six-day period, each muscle group gets a good, solid workout. The bad news is, for five days, that muscle group does not get a good, solid workout!

And this is where subgroups come into play. This will not be a lengthy chapter, but it is an important one, I think.

By the time a workout is done, the tendency is to give ourselves the, "Poor baby, you are so tired and sore; let's go rub some liniment on the muscles" routine.

Not so fast, cupcake. If you have time, there is one more thing to do.

I try my best at the end of each workout to do one more exercise set of a different muscle group than the one that I have been doing. On chest day, I will probably do shoulder press as well for 1-3 sets at the end of the routine. On biceps day, I will likely also do leg press or calf raises for 1-3 sets at the end of the routine. On triceps day, I will probably do biceps curls for 1-3 sets at the end of the routine. On back day, I will probably do bench press dumbbell presses for 1-3 sets at the end of the routine. On shoulders day, I will probably do triceps rope pulldown for 1-3 sets at the end of the routine. On leg day, I will probably do wide grip pull-ups for 1-3 sets at the end of the routine.

Think of it this way. It is kind of like reminding a muscle group that you have not forgotten about them. For me personally, I find that it keeps them fit and functional and progressing far more than if I only hit that muscle group one time a week.

Like I said, short but important chapter.

Section Three
Beyond The Workout

Chapter Eleven
Supplements: Friend or Foe?

Anyone who has been in the gym for a while has learned to spot them; the unnaturally huge, wild-eyed, short-tempered behemoths that have enough "juice" in their system to soak the desert and make it spring to life.

Back in the day, steroids were all the rage. The tide seems to be turning just a bit on that, mostly because people are starting to realize the physical damage it does to the entire body. But instead of the tide turning to only that which is safe and natural, the void has been filled with a great many other things that are dangerous in their own right.

I should tell you, at this point, that if you are waiting for me to give you the secret chemical recipe to make Arnold Schwarzennegar look tiny, then this is not the book for you.

Earlier today, as I write this (I am at a Christian summer camp), I received a public compliment that pleased me immeasurably: "I mean, Brother Wagner back there is jacked; we can all see that."

I smiled. Jacked is good.

And I have not done a single unnatural thing to get this way. Are there guys "more huger" than me? Absolutely. Do I care? Not if they have done something stupid to achieve that size, no. My goal is not to be the biggest human on the planet; my goal is to be healthy and strong and fit and active.

So, are supplements "friend or foe" in that pursuit?

The answer is, "That depends." Just like people can be friend or foe depending on who and what they are, supplements can also be friend or foe.

I have chosen to keep things very simple, and it has worked very well, I think. To me, there are only a handful of things needed to maximize your workout efforts.

Protein from your food.

High-quality protein is the holy grail of fitness and exercise. And the bulk of it needs to come from your diet. No, this is not a supplement; it is a staple. But I still want to mention it up front, because no good nutritional/exercise plan is complete without it. My favorite choices on this are non-fried chicken, cottage cheese, steak, and eggs. Grilled fish is excellent as well, but I am just not a big fan of fish. Protein is the main muscle builder for your body; it repairs and rebuilds muscle tissue that is broken down as you work out, making your muscles bigger and stronger along the way.

Good multivitamins.

It is at this point that many people are going to try to sell you their brand of special miracle vitamins that will build your muscles, improve your love life, give you fresh breath, and turn you into a concert pianist. I will do no such thing; I am not a vitamin salesman and do not ever intend to be.

My personal choice in multivitamins is the simple GNC Mega Men vitamins. I use the Sport edition. I have found that it gives me a solid energy boost throughout the day, which is really helpful in my workouts. And it is pretty cheap, too, which is always helpful.

Whey protein powder.

This is another staple of bodybuilding. It is a very natural product, the byproduct of the cheese-making process. Especially if you are trying to build muscle mass, it is an excellent way to get the high amount of protein your body will need for a day. And once again, I do not find the need to buy the expensive, famous-weight-lifter-approved protein powder that costs twice as much as the stuff you can get from Walmart or Amazon. As long as it is simple, natural whey protein powder, it will do nicely, thank you very much.

Creatine.

Creatine is one of the most widely studied supplements of the past four decades, and is widely regarded as very safe. It is a natural product; in fact, your own body produces it every single day. It is a nitrogenous organic acid that provides energy to the cells of your muscles, helping you to lift better and stronger as you work out. It also aids in muscle recovery after the workout. It helps the muscles to retain water, making them appear bigger and fuller. It is found naturally in red meat and in seafood. As a supplement, I take one of the provided scoops per day, every day.

That's it. That is my entire supplement list.

I have not said anything about pre-workout supplements, and you may find that a bit odd. So let me address that right now. I am not completely opposed to *safe and natural* pre-workout mixes. I just do not think many of them qualify as safe and natural, nor do I like the way they make me feel. I have yet to find any that do not make me jittery or itchy or give me headaches, so I personally normally avoid them. I have found that a cup of coffee or glass of tea, combined with my vitamins, generally gives me all the boost I need to lift well; so why add one more unnecessary thing?

Chapter Twelve
All Through the Day

The battle was over before it started, really; with 1410 soldiers on one side, and only 30 on the other, the outcome was never really in doubt. Mind you, the 30 fought valiantly; anyone watching would have been impressed with how hard they tried. But the numbers were simply far too stacked against them, and they had no chance to succeed.

Have you figured it out yet?

The soldiers represent minutes in a day. Each one of us is allotted 1440 of them for each new day. The 30 are the minutes even the most dedicated person normally spends working out each day. Therefore, the remaining 1410 are the minutes we do not spend working out.

I can almost hear you sucking in your breath, assuming that I am going to present some improbable, pie-in-the-sky platitude to correct and rework those numbers for you. But I am well aware that life is busy; we all spend most of our time working, a bunch of our time serving the Lord, and a bunch of time tending to our homes and families. Honestly, then, if you actually are getting in a half hour of exercise every day, you are probably doing far better than most!

But it still isn't enough. If you are going to be as fit and healthy as you can be, you will need to find some other way to change the dynamic that those numbers present. And that is where a philosophy that I call "all through the day" comes into play. In practical terms, it means that you need to be conscious of the choices that you make during the day and intentionally make choices that will get your body moving.

Here are some of the choices that I have found to be incredibly helpful to this "all through the day" philosophy.

Stairs are your friend.

As a pastor, I spend a lot of time during the average week making hospital visits, normally to the hospital in Shelby, North Carolina. The people I visit are almost always on the third floor or above, since the second floor is the birthing ward. Each and every time I go to the hospital, I breeze right past the elevator as if the devil himself lives inside; I know where the stairs are, and that is where I am headed.

The flights themselves are far longer than average, which is great. So I will go up 3 to 5 flights of stairs, then make my way back down the same 3 to 5 flights of stairs every time I go to the hospital. And I do not take them slow; I either run them or climb them very fast. By the time I get to the top, I always have to take a moment or so and pace back and forth and get my breathing back under control before making my visit.

Pick up the pace.

This is a line I repeat to myself many times a day. When I am walking out of the church to my vehicle (Which I intentionally park a decent way away from the building) or to the church from my vehicle, I remind myself, "Pick up the pace," and I speed my walking up to a very fast clip. I walk fast down the hallways. I walk fast from one building to the next, or actually run between them. Little bursts of intense activity like that during the day make more of a difference than you may realize!

Take a fit break.

Back in the day, it was incredibly popular for people to take "smoke breaks" at work. Folks normally laugh at that now, realizing how unhealthy it is—while they are shoving Twix and Snickers from the vending machine into their mouths as they stand around and do nothing.

To paraphrase Paul, "Behold, I show you a more excellent way..."

I take fit breaks during the day rather than smoking breaks or snacking breaks. Mind you, this is on my "desk days;" on the days when I am rebuilding my barn in the heat of the summer, or working on the church roof, they are not really necessary. But on any day that is even remotely sedentary, I do my best, three to four times a day, to get out from behind the desk and do five to seven minutes of intense activity. I may lift the weights that I have in my cabinet. I may do jumping jacks, push-ups, or burpees. I may run in place or do fast knee lifts or rebounds. I may do air squats or calf raises. But those fit breaks make a difference in my overall health and strength, and as a nice bonus, they get me revved back up and ready to work faster and better when I get back to the desk.

Take a stand.

Those words are not unfamiliar to a Christian, and especially not to a preacher. It is not a moral stand that I am referring to this moment, though, as I type these words. I am talking about choosing standing over sitting when it is possible, as you do your work. As I type this, I am actually standing at a table rather than sitting in a chair. I have been doing so for about the last hour. That is 60 minutes that I have been upright and moving my legs up and down rather than sitting and stagnating.

Take a walk.

Television and video games and doom scrolling on smartphones have become a normal part of the American day. But not only do they waste time, they also waste valuable opportunities during the day both to improve your health and improve your relationship with those that you love. Whenever Dana and I get to go home early enough for the sun to still be shining, we normally change right into our walking clothes and start heading down our road. Two and a half miles and forty minutes later, we are back home. We have spent precious time together talking, we have enjoyed the outdoors and the scenery, we have gotten a nice dose of vitamin D from the sun, and we have become that much more fit.

And now you know how to tip the scales on that 1410 to 30 daily battle.

Chapter Thirteen
Staying Fit on the Road

The contents of this chapter will not apply to everyone, but they will apply to a lot of the people that I know and love. And if you travel at all, all of this will definitely apply to you.

Life on the road is a very difficult thing, and I am very well acquainted with it. Mind you, I consider myself absolutely, utterly blessed. In addition to pastoring a spectacularly wonderful church, I get to do evangelistic meetings, youth camps, revivals, and other special meetings all over the country, and even in many countries around the world. Just in the past month, as I write this, I have been from Tennessee, to South Carolina, to Virginia, back to South Carolina, back to Tennessee, and now am in Virginia again.

Needless to say, trying to stay fit while being in so many different hotels that you often wake up wondering what state you are in is a challenge, to say the least. At home, I have my own personal gym, good food readily at hand, and a great deal of control over my schedule. On the road, there may or may not be a decent gym nearby, the hotel may or may not have a decent fitness room, and the food will either come through a window or be a lavish church spread high in deliciousness but low on helpfulness.

What is a health-conscious person to do?

Let me walk you through it.

To begin with, make up your mind that you are going to work out every single day, even if it is only in your hotel room.

It can be done; if you give me a patch of floor six feet long and three feet wide, I can do a full workout. That is sometimes necessary; sometimes, but nowhere near always. Most hotels do, in fact, have a fitness room. And even if they do not have much in the way of weights, they do provide space, and you can provide the rest. If you do not care to spend a bit of money, though, usually $10 a day, most any decent gym will allow you to buy a guest pass and work out. Most will also cut you a good deal for the entire week.

Is none of that available? Then go for a hike, a walk, or a run. On a mission trip to St. Lucia, I ran back and forth to the beach every day, going through neighborhood after neighborhood, figuring out my way as I went. Whenever Dana and I are in Georgia or Tennessee or Virginia, we are almost certainly going to be hiking during the day.

Invest in good, portable equipment that you can carry with you in your travels.

Directly in front of me as I write this, I am staring at my portable Finer Form weight bench. It has folding legs, making it easy to carry with me most anywhere I go. Off to my left, I am looking at my 50-pound adjustable dumbbells that I also brought with me to camp. With just those two things, I will be able to get a very decent workout every single day that I am here without ever having to leave the camp.

Weight bands (be sure and check out the videos on those from Pastor Chris Hewett) are another excellent choice, and take up very little space in a suitcase.

Buy a good cooler, and bring your healthy foods with you.

We splurged and bought a Yeti cooler. It has been money well spent; it keeps our grapes and plums and cheese and cherries and veggies and other helpful things cool and fresh for a very long time wherever we go.

I bring bottles of unsweet tea with me. Dana brings bottles of water. We have no excuse to binge on candy and potato chips on the road, because we have better options with us.

Choose the best options for each situation.

With as many miles as we travel and as tight as our schedule is, it is inevitable that a great deal of our food is going to be handed to us through a window. And yet, even there, there are some choices that are markedly healthier than others. At Wendy's, I will be getting the baked potato instead of French fries. Wherever we go, I will be seeking out the grilled chicken rather than anything that is fried. If a side salad or seasonal fruit is an option, I will be choosing those.

At church dinners, I will be looking for whatever is grilled, avoiding white, fluffy rolls and breads, loading up on fruits and vegetables, and taking "sample-sized portions" of any desserts I choose to indulge in.

All of this takes work, preparation, and dedication. But "death by traveling" is just as final as "death by giving the leader of the Hells Angels a wedgie."

Chapter Fourteen
Intermittent Fasting

And now, dear reader, I turn you over to two more dear friends, Wesley and Carrie Morrison, for a discussion on Intermittent Fasting. Though I do not use it, I have seen it work wonders for them, and I knew you would benefit from their perspective and insight. Bo Wagner.

In the fall of 2021, Carrie and I picked up a book called Fast, Feast, Repeat by Gin Stephens—and without exaggeration, it changed our lives.

We weren't hunting for a new diet. Like many people, we had tried them all: low-fat, low-carb, calorie counting, journaling, point systems, shakes, supplements, fads. And like most people, we were burned out and quietly skeptical. Even when we lost weight, we couldn't keep it off. It felt like we were constantly at war with our own plates. But what Fast, Feast, Repeat introduced us to wasn't just a new plan—it was a new mindset, a simple, sustainable, science-backed lifestyle known as intermittent fasting (or IF). And it made more sense than anything we'd ever tried.

From Diets to Discipline

Intermittent fasting isn't about what you eat. It's about when you eat. That single sentence changed everything for us. Instead of obsessing over macros or eliminating our favorite foods, we simply began narrowing our eating window each day. For example, with an 18/6 approach, we fasted for 18 hours and ate during a 6-hour window that worked best for our daily schedule.

That's it. No pills. No complicated charts. No shame if we wanted a cheeseburger now and then.

We were stunned to discover this truth: within our eating window, we weren't bound by rigid food rules. There were no forbidden foods or complicated formulas. Just real-life flexibility that felt doable. And not only did it work—it felt right. Within three months, we had lost a combined 40 pounds. But more importantly, we felt better than we had in years. Our energy levels climbed. Our focus improved. Our lab results got better. And our grocery bills got lower. Plus, with fewer meals to prep, clean, and plan, we suddenly had more time in our day—something that mattered greatly with our full-time ministry schedule.

We also began to see unexpected personal health breakthroughs. Carrie was able to come off her blood pressure medication completely. And our middle daughter, who had struggled with stubborn acne for years—despite countless visits to the dermatologist—saw her skin completely clear up after adopting IF.

Why It Works: The Benefits of Intermittent Fasting

Based on current research, here are some of the possible health benefits of intermittent fasting:
• Weight Management and Metabolic Health.
• Weight Loss: IF can help reduce calorie intake and boost fat burning.
• Improved Insulin Sensitivity and Reduced Risk of Type 2 Diabetes.
• Enhanced Fat Burning: Promotes the breakdown of stored fat.
• Metabolic Flexibility: Helps your body switch between glucose and fat for fuel.
• Heart Health.
• Improved Blood Pressure.
• Improved Cholesterol Levels: May reduce LDL and triglycerides.
• Reduced Risk of Heart Disease through better blood markers and inflammation.

- Brain Health.
- Improved Thinking and Memory.
- Protection Against Neurodegenerative Diseases like Alzheimer's and Parkinson's

(animal studies).

- Cellular and Other Benefits:
- Cellular Repair and Autophagy: Removes waste materials from cells.
- Reduced Inflammation.
- Potential Cancer Prevention and Treatment Support (animal studies).
- Improved Gut Health: Positive influence on gut microbiome.
- Possible Increased Longevity (in animal models).

Important Note: Always consult a healthcare professional before starting intermittent fasting, especially if you are pregnant, breastfeeding, managing medical conditions, or taking medications. IF may not be suitable for everyone.

Turning Practice into Ministry

As we experienced the benefits firsthand, we couldn't help but share what we'd learned.

The results sparked a lot of curiosity among our friends and family. One question led to another, and before long, we found ourselves having the same conversations over and over.

So we did something simple: we started a Facebook group. There was nothing to buy. No product to push. Just a place to share our story, encourage others, answer questions, and keep it real. And to our surprise, the group grew quickly. People weren't just curious, they were hungry for something real. Something that worked. Something sustainable. We did live Q&A sessions, answered common questions, and shared both our victories and our struggles. And over time, that little community became a place where real change happened.

Real Talk: IF Isn't Magic

Let's be honest: intermittent fasting isn't magic. It takes commitment. If you're sipping flavored lattes during your fast or using your eating window as a daily excuse to binge, it is not going to work.

Some people want change without changing. But lasting transformation—physical or Spiritual—requires intentionality. IF isn't a shortcut. But it is the most sustainable lifestyle we have ever found, and is simple, Biblical, and free.

In a world that complicates everything, intermittent fasting reminds us that freedom is often found in simplicity. And self-discipline is still one of the greatest paths to peace. If you are on the fence, we urge you to try it. Not for a weekend. Not for a quick fix. But for 30 to 60 days. Be consistent. Be honest. And give your body and mind time to adjust. We believe you'll be glad you did.

Getting Started with IF: A Quick Guide

1. Choose Your Eating Window: Start with something like 18:6 (e.g., 1:00 PM to 7:00 PM).
Find a window that fits your life.
2. Keep the Fast Clean: Only consume plain water, black coffee (no cream or sweeteners), and unsweetened tea during your fasting window.
3. Hydrate, Hydrate, Hydrate: Aim to drink at least half your body weight in ounces of water daily (e.g., 160 lbs = 80 oz).
4. Don't Obsess Over What You Eat: Eat real meals during your window. Over time, your cravings may shift toward healthier choices.
5. Trust the Process: The first week or two may be hard. But stick with it—change comes with consistency.

Frequently Asked Questions

- Q: Can I really eat anything I want?
- A: Technically, yes. But IF isn't a license to overeat junk food. Most people naturally eat better the longer they fast consistently.
- Q: What can I eat or drink during the fast?
- A: Water (plain), black coffee, and unsweetened tea. That's it. Even a splash of cream breaks the fast.
- Q: Will I be hungry all the time?
- A: Maybe at first, but hunger fades as your body adapts. Hunger comes in waves—and passes.
- Q: What if I mess up or eat outside my window?
- A: Don't quit! Just start again at your next fast. Progress, not perfection.
- Q: How soon will I see results?
- A: Some people see results in the first few weeks. Others take longer. Focus on the process, not just the scale.
- Q: Is fasting biblical?
- A: Yes! Fasting appears throughout Scripture as a spiritual discipline and a way to draw closer to God.
- Q: Is this safe long-term?
- A: For most healthy individuals, yes. But check with your doctor if you have medical conditions or take medications.

Final Thought

We believe IF is one of the most powerful tools the Lord has allowed us to use—for our health, our marriage, our ministry, and our mindset. It's brought clarity, peace, and margin.

If our journey encourages you to begin your own, then praise the Lord. We're cheering you on.

Wesley & Carrire Morrison

Chapter Fifteen
Don't Let the Stuff You Have Kill You

It was a horror scene that a Hollywood producer would envy. No one knows exactly how it happened; they just know that Rick never saw it coming. He walked into his house after work like any other day, took a few steps inside the door—and was rudely ambushed. He could feel his head reeling from the blow as his body tumbled to the floor. Someone had struck him in the head from behind, clearly intent on ending his life. Instinctively, Rick rolled over onto his back and into a defensive position. But that is when his eyes grew wide as if he was seeing an unspeakable terror; his refrigerator, that long faithful friend, was leaning over him, glaring, ready to dive on him and crush him to death.

Rick threw his legs up, catching it in the mid-section as it dove down on him. Like some cowboy from an old black and white movie, he pushed upward with all his might and sent the refrigerator flipping over his head and away from him. But as he rolled up onto one knee to continue the fight, he was rammed in the side and sent reeling yet again. What fresh new enemy had joined this lethal fight against him? As Rick caught his breath and whirled back around to face this new foe, he found himself face to face with his kitchen cabinets.

Two doors swung open, one from either side, smashing into his ears. He winced in pain, but determined not to succumb, threw a hard uppercut into the bottom of the cabinet, breaking it pretty badly...

The end.

Ahem. I assume you know that the above fight did not really happen. And yet, people's refrigerators and cabinets often are, in fact, trying to kill them. I suppose it would be more proper and accurate, though, to say that what people put into those refrigerators and cabinets is trying to kill them. And that makes the entire affair their own fault, not the fault of the appliance or the cabinet.

Do you know what ends up in your refrigerator and cabinets? Whatever you put there, no more, and no less. And that makes it inexcusable that most people are importing their own culinary demise.

I hate to waste money. I suppose it would be more accurate to say that I HAAAATTTTTEEE to waste money. And yet, sometimes that is going to be necessary for the greater good. If you really want to get fit and healthy, there is going to have to come a point in time when you get absolutely ruthless with what you already have in your refrigerator and cabinets and ruthless about making sure that it changes for the long term, not for the moment. How in the world do people ever expect to get fit and healthy when their cabinets are loaded with unhealthy snacks, candy, candy bars, processed foods, Little Debbie's, Twinkies, oatmeal cakes, potato chips, Doritos, white bread, the list could go on and on forever.

You likely need to throw a bunch of stuff out and start over. The average kid is already doomed from childhood, because their parents have loaded the house up with snacks that are designed to fatten the kids up like they are being prepared for the oven of Hansel and Gretel's witch.

You will eat what you have. You will not eat what you do not have.

Let me repeat that: You will eat what you have. You will not eat what you do not have.

Why do kids grow up with an insatiable sweet tooth for horrible things? Mostly because that is what was always most readily available to them. Why do adults continue that trend? Mostly because that is what is always most readily available to them.

So change that. Have a kitchen and pantry cleaning day in which you throw out the vast bulk of the stuff that is tasty but horrible, and replace it with stuff that is tasty and helpful. Make sure you have whole wheat, sourdough, or some other mostly healthy bread rather than white bread. Make sure you have fresh fruits and vegetables handy instead of packaged junk snacks. Go through everything, weed out the unhealthy, and replace it with the healthy.

Refrigerators and cabinets make wonderful servants, but terrifying monsters.

Chapter Sixteen
Your Fitness Affects Your Finances

One last bit of motivation to get all of this done before we go. I have written at length about exercise and nutrition. But I have also been honest that it takes work, effort, and discipline to actually do all of this. And, especially as we covered the last two chapters, I encouraged you both to invest in good workout equipment and to throw out a bunch of unhealthy food and replace it with healthy food.

Those two things cost money. Because of that, many people automatically determine that "they cannot afford to do all of that." So, please allow me to provide you with a bit of perspective if I may. Below is a list of the average per-person cost of a few things, all of which are commonly caused by obesity:

Treatment for a heart attack - $100,000
Treatment for heart disease (per year) - $5,500
Treatment for a stroke - $140,000
Treatment for diabetes (per year) - $19,000
Treatment for high blood pressure (per year) - $2,800
Treatment for high cholesterol (per year) - $15,000
Treatment for sleep apnea (per year) - $2,100
Treatment for kidney disease (per year) - $50,000
Treatment for gallstones - $20,000
Treatment for osteoarthritis (lifetime) - $20,000
Treatment for colon cancer - $50,000
Treatment for atherosclerosis - $20,000

I could add a great many more expensive and debilitating things to this list, but I think you get the point. Anyone saying "I cannot afford to get fit!" is a million miles (and maybe a million dollars) off base. The fact is, you cannot afford *not to get fit*. And I did not even deal with the costs of long-term in-home care, nursing homes, rehab facilities, and many other expensive things people have to pay for many, many long years before they should have, if ever!

I have teased my children for years that, one day, I will come to visit them in their nursing homes. Anything could happen, and James 4:14 has taught me well never to assume or presume, but it is my genuine goal to live healthy and independent until I get so very old that I die peacefully in my sleep at home, leaving my enemies to say, "Finally! I thought that old coot was going to live forever!"

And a nice bonus to being healthy and not incurring all of those unneeded costs I listed above is that I can spend my money on more pleasant things like cruises, excursions, adventures, and making our home nicer and nicer, and I can also invest in things that will make my family better and better off. I also have more to give to the church and to missions and to those in need.

You can do it—and you can't afford not to.

Chapter Seventeen
Getting Fit Despite Severe Limitations

It was an eye-opening, yet really cool request. A dear lady who has watched many of my workout videos online contacted me and Dana to ask for advice. She has been on a fitness and health journey of her own and has done a pretty good job of it. But she has difficulty with her knees, and as such, there are many exercises that I recommend for legs that she cannot do. She wanted to know if there were any exercises for the legs that she could do that would keep her knees out of it. In pretty short order, I wrote back and gave her a list and descriptions of all of them.

That conversation got me thinking, though. Much of what I have recommended by way of working out presupposes that people have the basic physical ability needed to do so. They can stand, bend down, raise up, lift, etc. So, is there any hope for those who have severe limitations, either of their own making or through no fault of their own?

The answer, in most cases, is yes.

Let's start with the absolute basics.

Your body is your ally in this, even though you may not realize it. As you sit there thinking, "I cannot do anything at all to burn calories!" do you know what you have been doing?

Burning calories.

You, sir or madam, are never totally inactive unless you are dead. You breathe around 25,000 times per day. Your heart beats 100,000 or so times per day. You blink around 19,000 times per day. You sneeze about four times per day. You cough eighteen or so times per day. You swallow roughly 600 times per day. You say roughly 16,000 words per day. In other words, just existing as a living being takes calories, lots of them. Every time you lift your hand or wiggle your foot or shake your head, you are burning calories. Every time you smile or frown, you are burning calories. You will burn calories every single day that you live, without exception. And this means that even if you are morbidly obese and in a wheelchair (in which case, you really should see a doctor), you still have an enormous amount of control over whether you ultimately get fit. In the most basic sense, it boils down to eating fewer calories than your body is burning, and doing so over a long period of time.

If I woke up tomorrow and found that I had somehow gained 400 pounds overnight, was wheelchair bound, and could not even fit through the gym door, the first words out of my mouth would be "AAAAGGGGGHHHHHHH WHAT HAPPENED?!?" But the very next words out of my mouth would be "Bring me water and celery for lunch." I would be fixated on making sure that I ate several hundred fewer calories per day than my now-sedentary body was burning. If I could do nothing else, that all by itself would almost certainly begin to make the pounds melt off.

Beyond that, a person with severe limitations should ask themselves this one question: "What can I move?"

A friend of mine was paralyzed from the waist down. He was also determined to be healthy. He wheeled himself into the gym each day and worked upper body: chest, biceps, triceps, shoulders, lats. From the waist up, he was absolutely ripped. He knew what he could move, so he moved it.

If you, for whatever reason, are unable to stand, pick up something with your hands and start working out. Soup can? Yes, that will work. Hammer? Even better. A big, heavy Bible? Curl it, read it, then curl it some more; let it improve your weak soul and your weak body. Every movement you make engages a muscle group and burns calories, no exceptions.

You say, "But I am in a wheelchair; I can't do cardio like others, so what does it matter?"

What do you mean you can't do cardio? Do you know how good a cardio workout you can get by wheeling yourself around at top speed? You can get a cardio workout that a person with two good legs would be envious of!

Move. Just move!

Your problem may be far less severe, but a problem nonetheless. Like the lady I mentioned at the beginning of this chapter, maybe you just have serious joint issues. If so, you should still be eating right, and you should still be moving; you just need to remember the words "low impact." Think something like pool aerobics or swimming. Think of exercises that isolate muscles apart from the joints that hurt. For the lady asking about legs, I recommended the abductor and adductor machines. I also recommended simple chair exercises that, though they sound easy, really do help.

Try sitting in a chair with your feet flat on the floor, then, keeping them bent the way they are, pulling them upward as high as you can, holding them at the top of the movement for a second, then slowly lowering them. Your knees are just along for the ride; your quadriceps are doing the work. For calves, a person with knee issues can usually use a seated calf machine. The weight is resting on the lower quads, and the knees are again mostly along for the ride as you lift from the calves.

Think through each muscle you can move, find ways to isolate hurting joints out of the lifting, and go to it.

Chapter Eighteen
A Word Before I Go

You can do this. I know, I know, you have heard me say that throughout the book. But it really is true; you can do this. If you are reading this book, you are obviously still alive and sentient. That being the case, you can still move, even if it is just to nod your head, and you still have control over what you put in your mouth.

As you go through your fitness journey, don't be discouraged. It is oftentimes painfully slow, but the body responds as God designed it to respond. Furthermore, since your body is the temple of the Holy Ghost, God has a vested interest in helping you to keep that temple in as good condition as it can be. So make it a matter of prayer. Don't just push, pray. Don't just pull, pray. Bring God into this, apologize for letting yourself go, and set about changing things for the better.

And would you do one or two more things, please, things that would mean a great deal to me? If you get help from this book, please let me know (you can email me at 2knowhim.bw@gmail.com) so that I can rejoice with you and cheer you on; I really want it to make a difference in your life. Please let others know about this book as well; if it helped you, it could help others as well. And if you would leave the book a good rating and review on Amazon, I would appreciate that as well.

God bless you, and you can do this!

Other Books by Dr. Wagner

Colossians: The Treasure of Deity
Daniel: Breathtaking
Ephesians: The Treasures of Family
Esther: Five Feasts and the Fingerprints of God
Galatians: The Treasures of Liberty
Hosea: Love When It Matters Most
James: The Pen and the Plumb Line
Joel, Amos, Obadiah: Turmoil Among the Nations
Jonah: A Story of Greatness
Nehemiah: A Labor of Love
Philippians: The Treasures of Joy
Proverbs Vol 1: Bright Light from Dark Sayings
Proverbs Vol 2: Bright Light from Dark Sayings
The Revelation: Ready or Not
Romans: Salvation from A-Z
Ruth: Diamonds in the Darkness

Beyond the Colored Coat
From Footers to Finish Nails
Learning Not to Fear the Old Testament
Marriage Makers/Marriage Breakers
I'm Saved! Now What???
Don't Muzzle the Ox
Why Christmas?

Books in the Night Heroes Series

Cry from the Coal Mine (Vol 1)
Free Fall (Vol 2)
Broken Brotherhood (Vol 3)
The Blade of Black Crow (Vol 4)

Ghost Ship (Vol 5)
When Serpents Rise (Vol 6)
Moth Man (Vol 7)
Runaway (Vol 8)
Terror by Day (Vol 9)
Winter Wolf (Vol 10)
Desert Heat (Vol 11)
Deadline (Vol 12)
The Sword and the Iron Curtain (Vol 13)
Escape From Beaver Island (Vol 14)

Other Fiction

Zak Blue: Falcon Wing
Zak Blue: Enter the Maelstrom

Devotionals

DO Drops Vol. 1
DO Drops Vol. 2
DO Drops Vol. 3
DO Drops Vol. 4
DO Drops Vol. 5
DO Drops Vol. 6
DO Drops Vol. 7
DO Drops Vol. 8
DO Drops Vol. 9
DO Drops Vol. 10
DO Drops Vol. 11
DO Drops Vol. 12
DO Drops Vol. 13

www.ingramcontent.com/pod-product-compliance
Lightning Source LLC
Chambersburg PA
CBHW072131270326
41931CB00010B/1722